Medicine in
the Old West

Medicine in the Old West

A History, 1850–1900

Jeremy Agnew

McFarland & Company, Inc., Publishers

Jefferson, North Carolina, and London

LIBRARY OF CONGRESS CATALOGUING-IN-PUBLICATION DATA

Agnew, Jeremy.
   Medicine in the Old West : a history, 1850–1900 /
Jeremy Agnew.
      p.   cm.
   Includes bibliographical references and index.

   ISBN 978-0-7864-4623-0
   softcover : 50# alkaline paper ∞

   1. Medicine—West (U.S.)—History—19th century.
2. West (U.S.)—History—19th century.   I. Title.
R154.5.W47A34   2010
610.978—dc22   2010009297

British Library cataloguing data are available

Front cover: Typical Denver office at the turn of the century with
a doctor (thought to be L.F. Preston) administering an injection
(©2010 Colorado Historical Society, Buckwalter Collection);
ornaments ©2010 clipart.com

Manufactured in the United States of America

McFarland & Company, Inc., Publishers
  Box 611, Jefferson, North Carolina 28640
    www.mcfarlandpub.com

To the memory of my grandfather,
Samuel Foskett, M.D.,
who inspired in me an interest in medical matters
that has lasted throughout the years

Contents

Chronology of Medical Developments in the Old West

1796   Edward Jenner uses cowpox to vaccinate against smallpox

1800   Average life expectancy is 34½ years for men and 36½ for women

1816   Rudimentary stethoscope invented

1820   Quinine isolated in France from the bark of the *chinchona* tree

1831   Chloroform developed; used initially for recreational inhalation

1839   Vulcanization of India rubber by Charles Goodyear leads to the development of rubber condoms and hygiene syringes, and the use of vulcanite for false teeth

1841   First small group of pioneers sets out across Kansas along the Oregon Trail

1842   William Clarke uses ether as an anesthetic for a tooth extraction; Crawford Long of Georgia uses ether for minor operations

1848   First news of the gold strike at Sutter's Mill in California; end of the Mexican War adds parts of Texas and California to the United States

1849   Transcontinental gold rush of Forty-Niners to the California gold camps

1850   Ignatz Semmelweiss announces that childbed fever infections are transmitted by doctors

1854   Grattan Massacre in Wyoming sparks war with the Plains Indians for the next 36 years

1858   Development of the hypodermic syringe for direct injection through the skin into body tissue

1859   Major gold rushes to Central City, Colorado, and Bannack, Montana.

1860   Start of the Pony Express; average life expectancy is 41 years for men and 43 years for women

1861   Start of the Civil War between the Union and the Confederates; completion of the transcontinental telegraph and end of the Pony Express

1862   Louis Pasteur shows that bacteria are the cause of fermentation

1865   End of the Civil War

1866   First herd of Texas cattle heads up the Sedalia Trail to meet the railroad in Kansas

1867   Joseph Lister uses carbolic acid in antiseptic surgery; Thomas Allbutt develops the modern type of clinical thermometer

1869   Completion of the transcontinental railroad links the East to California

1870   Beginning of the worst years of warfare with the Plains Indians

1874   Synthesis of heroin, considered to be a non-addictive substitute for morphine

1876   Custer's defeat at the Battle of the Little Bighorn; Robert Koch identifies the bacteria that cause anthrax

1878   Robert Koch discovers the bacteria that cause infection of wounds

1879   Albert Neisser discovers the bacteria that causes gonorrhea.

1880   The parasite that causes malaria is discovered

1881   The Gunfight at the OK Corral in Tombstone, Arizona

1882   Robert Koch isolates the bacillus that causes tuberculosis

1883   Modern type of rubber contraceptive diaphragm developed by German physiologist C. Hasse (Wilhelm Mensinga); Robert Koch discovers the organism that causes cholera

1884   Carl Koller uses cocaine as a local anesthetic for eye operations

1885   Essential end of the cattle drives from Texas, and the Kansas cowtown era; Pasteur develops successful vaccination against rabies

1890   End of the Indian Wars after the fight at Wounded Knee, South Dakota; William Halsted introduces the use of rubber gloves for surgery

1895   Discovery of x-rays allows physicians and surgeons to see inside a patient; development of acetylsalicylic acid (better known as aspirin) by Bayer Company in Germany

1897   Discovery by Ronald Ross that the malaria parasite is transmitted by the *Anopheles* mosquito.

1900   Average life expectancy is 48 years for men and 51 years for women

1901   Walter Reed and colleagues prove the role of the mosquito in the spread of yellow fever; organization of the Military Dental Corps

1905   Fritz Schaudinn and Erich Hoffman discover the spirochete that causes syphilis

1910   Salvarsan 606 is announced as a cure for syphilis by Paul Ehrlich in Germany

1928   The antibiotic penicillin is discovered by Alexander Fleming (but not produced in quantity until 1939)

1945   Start of the widespread use of penicillin

Preface

We live today in an age of modern medical miracles. It is easy to forget, however, that 90 percent of "modern" medicine dates from after World War II.

This book is a history of the healing arts as practiced in the Old West between approximately 1850 and 1900. The theme of the book broadly covers the perils to health that were present during the expansion of the American frontier, and the methods used by doctors to overcome them. Whether the challenge was sickness, an Indian arrow, a gunshot wound, or a fall from a horse, the victim was often far from medical care and had to make do until he or she could reach a doctor. Medical treatment was often primitive, and diseases that today we take for granted as curable were often fatal. Without today's understanding of the basis for disease, physicians could often only provide supportive care and hope that patients recovered by themselves.

The reader will note, as a recurrent theme, the obsession of early frontier medicine with emptying the bowels through laxatives, purgative drugs, and enemas. This idea, which was rooted in Greek medicine, was prominent through the nineteenth century as a generic treatment to expel disease by emptying the system. This obsession continued, in diminished form, through much of the twentieth century—certainly up to the 1970s.

My interest in medicine was sparked while I was growing up with my grandfather, an English Victorian–era doctor who practiced "frontier medicine" in India in the early 1900s. From him I first heard of such mysterious nineteenth-century maladies as "bilious attacks," "catarrh," "morbid excitement," "conniption fits," and other vague terms that were still being used to describe illnesses. My grandfather was invalided back to England after contracting malaria in India. At that time malaria was still basically incurable, and I remember him having recurrent attacks of fever when the *plasmodium* parasite in his system entered a new cycle. My grandfather continued to practice as a country doctor in Yorkshire, England, and I often accompanied him on his rounds to outlying farms and villages. One of his favorite cure-alls

1

was a pill that was a mixture of aspirin, phenacetin (acetophenetidin, a pain reliever), and caffeine.

My grandfather also started my lifelong love of the American West. Every Wednesday and Saturday he took the family to see a double feature at the movies. My grandfather's first choice was either a western or a musical. He would be delighted when both were on the same bill. I still love both genres.

As I grew older, I realized that motion pictures presented only one stylized and idealized view of the Old West. As I delved into history, however, I found that the real Old West was different but just as fascinating. My specific interest in medicine in the Old West as a comprehensive subject was sparked while doing research for two other books. I realized that disease, accidents, deliberate gunshot wounds, and how pioneers dealt with them played a large part in the lives of settlers, soldiers, and gunfighters. While trying to track down information for my other research, I realized that there was not a single comprehensive source that I could use. I continued to research and study the subject, and this book is the outcome.

When researching history, it is sometimes difficult to sort facts from errors, and correct dates from wrong ones, in source material. I have done my best to verify everything in this book with multiple sources, but in the end, I have to take the blame for any errors that have crept into the text.

CHAPTER ONE

Medicine from Mid-Century

In 1800 the average life expectancy for a man was thirty-four-and-a-half years, for a woman, thirty-six-and-a-half years. In 1860 it was forty-one years for men and forty-three years for women. By 1900 this had risen to forty-eight years for men and fifty-one years for women.

During the first half of the nineteenth century, medicine was still in a primitive state. Many babies died at birth, and many more succumbed to disease before they were five years old. Many mothers died in childbirth. Surgery was the same as it had been fifty years before, methods of performing operations were primitive, most sickness was treated at home, hospitals were rarely used, and the training of doctors was basic. Vaccines for common illnesses had not yet been developed. Surgery was hazardous due to a lack of anesthetics and lack of attention to infectious conditions.

As one example of misguided medical thinking, hydrocephalus involved an abnormal accumulation of fluid on the brain in children. Then called dropsy of the brain, the disease was thought to be produced by trying to excessively stimulate a child's intellect. One of the cures was to shave the child's head, then cover it with a poultice of onions stewed in vinegar. This disease, of course, is now known to be a result of interference with normal fluid circulation in the brain, caused by conditions such as tissue malformation, injury, infection, or a brain tumor.

The concepts of preventative medicine were not known. People were concerned with illness only after it happened, and physicians were expected to restore health rather than to preserve it. Surgery was primarily limited to amputation of damaged extremities, sewing up cuts, and splinting minor broken bones. Hospitals were viewed as places to die, not places to get well.

Pioneers and working men in the Old West commonly had to put up with scurvy, weariness, various aches and pains, numbness of limbs, swollen legs, blisters, bad breath, irritated gums, and loose teeth. Sickness, pain, and growing prematurely old was the lot they had to look forward to. The germs that caused typhus, dysentery, pneumonia, and miscellaneous fevers were

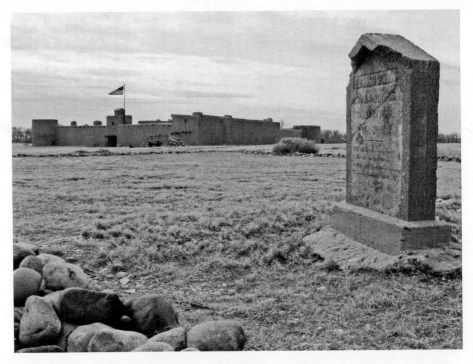

Stagecoach driver Edward Dorris died on the Santa Fe Trail in 1865 and was buried in this small cemetery at Bents Fort in Colorado (author's collection).

everywhere. The microorganisms responsible for these diseases found ideal conditions in concentrations of people, such as in cattle towns, mining camps, or wagon trains, so that they could spread and thrive among susceptible individuals.

The major trails for wagon trains headed west during the California gold rush were littered with graves, often recording cholera as the cause of death. Though most of the pioneers were young, all of them suffered frequently from dyspepsia and constipation due to poor diet and dehydration; rheumatism from sleeping out in cold, wet weather; and frequent injuries due to a hard outdoor life. Death caused by wild and domestic animals was common, and so were broken bones, bruises, and wounds due to extremes in the weather, hostile Indians, fires, and floods. Most cures were simple in concept. The recommended cure for a headache might be to bleed the patient, give him or her a cathartic, pour cold water on the head, and send the sufferer to bed.

The pioneers traveling to the West took what limited medical knowledge they had with them and learned to make do. Accidents, drowning, and gunshot wounds were leading causes of death and situations that required medical attention on the trail west. Most wagon trains did not have a doctor traveling with them, but wagon masters, out of necessity, had some limited medical knowledge. One source of pioneer medical information was recipe books of the mid-nineteenth century, which contained remedies for pain and fever (some of which were based on herbal remedies), and other simple medical procedures. The *Ladies' Indispensible Assistant*, for example, published in 1852, served some pioneers as the family physician, recommending treatments for diverse ailments such as cholera, smallpox, and dropsy. A multipurpose volume, it also contained instructions on how to perform vaccination for smallpox at home, along with recipes for food, stitching instructions, how to dye garments, and recommendations on etiquette.

A typical emigrant wagon train took along a medicine chest that included bandages, quinine, opium, whiskey, laxatives (often called "physicking pills"), splints, ammonia, castor oil, laudanum, sulfur pills, and morphine. They probably also included poultices of red pepper and mustard.

Death from disease in the Old West was typically due to infections from typhoid, yellow fever, diphtheria, malaria, measles, tuberculosis, cholera, and dysentery. Deaths from typhus and typhoid were particularly common due to overcrowding and poor sanitary conditions in many early camps and towns. Deaths from cancer or heart disease were uncommon because very few lived long enough for those diseases to develop to a fatal stage. Indeed, the incidence of lung cancer in the United States was rare before cigarette smoking became widespread.

During the nineteenth century the industrialization of the United States and the resulting mass movement of people from rural areas to work in factories in the cities brought with it an increase in the spread of common diseases. People living on widespread farms in rural areas of the West typically were not exposed to measles, mumps, chicken pox, scarlet fever, and other similar common childhood illnesses.

Diagnosis of diseases was haphazard due to a lack of understanding of disease mechanisms, and a lack of diagnostic instruments and today's sophisticated laboratory tests. Major diagnostic indicators were the pulse, skin color, breathing pattern, and color of a patient's urine. Diseases such as measles were diagnosed by smell. Diabetes was diagnosed by smelling the patient's breath or tasting a drop of his urine for sweetness.

As one example of the haphazard nature of frontier diagnostic accuracy, Arthur Hertzler, who later himself became a frontier physician, remembered that when he was a youth he went to a doctor after suffering a series of severe back pains that radiated into his groin. The doctor solemnly diagnosed that he was growing too fast. After a number of months of suffering, Hertzler passed a kidney stone.[1]

In 1861 the concept of germs and microbes had not yet been accepted.

Diagnosis of disease might be as vague as "inflammation of the chest," "inflammation of the bowels," or "suffered from a conniption fit." For example, in the 1830s people believed that cholera was a disease that attacked those who weakened themselves by overeating, intemperance, and similar sinful habits. Similarly, physicians did not know the cause of scurvy and attributed it to intemperance or sleeping in the cold. If a patient died, the true cause of death was often unknown, and death certificates might contain phrases such as "evil in the bladder" or the mysterious-sounding ailment called "effects of the jiggers."

In early Denver a man named Albert Cass was shot and killed in a saloon. His killer later died in jail, and the cause of death was listed as the "jim-jams." Doctors often could not make an accurate diagnosis of death because autopsies were considered to be sacrilegious and generally not performed.

In many instances "cures" were effected through folk remedies administered at home. Turpentine was used on aching joints. It might be mixed with lard to produce an ointment to treat a sore throat. Poultices were popular, and might be made from bread, onions, flaxseed, salt, or mustard. A mixture of sulfur, molasses, and cream of tartar was used "to purify the blood." Sassafras tea was used to "thin the blood" in order to withstand the heat of summer.

Though some of these remedies sound bizarre, some did have a basis in common sense and could assist the natural healing process. For example, cobwebs or wood ashes placed on a wound could reduce excessive bleeding by speeding clotting of the blood. Old Man's Beard, a web-like lichen that grows on pine trees, was used for the same purpose. The white of an egg applied to a burn would provide a protective cover for raw skin. The mold scraped into a wound from cheese that had turned green may have contained some antibiotic material that did resist infection and assisted healing.

Among the more dubious of the home remedies on the farm or ranch involved wounds, snakebite, or infection being treated with something as simple as a poultice made with tobacco or cow manure. Another dubious claim was that snails and earthworms mashed into a paste with water would cure diphtheria. One folk cure-all was composed of a combination of cow urine and dung.

The Theory of Humors

The basis for this state of medicine was a lack of advancement in medical science. In the mid–1800s, physicians were still being taught and using the humoral system that came from the ancient Greek physicians in 450 B.C. The basic concept was that there were four bodily fluids, called humors. These were blood (sanguis), phlegm (pituita), yellow bile (chole), and black bile (melanchole), which originated in the heart, brain, liver, and spleen respectively. These qualities corresponded to the four material elements of air, water, fire, and earth. The elements were a result of combining the fundamental qualities of hot, wet, cold, and dry. Blood, for example, was thought to make the body hot and wet, while black bile was considered to make it cold and dry, and phlegm made it cold and wet. The humors were thought to be responsible for body characteristics, such as body weight and the amount of hair. The manner in which the color of each humor was combined was also thought to be responsible for skin color, and made different people red or yellow, swarthy or pale.

Good health was thought to depend on an optimum balance of the four humors. For example, physicians felt that too much phlegm led to fevers and a runny nose. Too much black bile supposedly brought on "hypochondrial melancholy," a male psychological disease that was a result of Victorian man's supposed intellectual superiority over women.

Classical medicine based a "cure" for disease on reducing an excess of troublesome humors or impure fluids by expelling them from the body. The release of vomited material, diarrhea, and pus oozing from wounds was seen as evidence of the body ridding itself of putrid material. The extension of this thinking was that if these events could be forced to occur, then the doctor would be putting the patient back on the road to health.

Bleed, Purge, and Blister

Efforts to restore the balance in the humors subjected the patient to a series of treatments involving bleeding, purging, blistering, vomiting, and sweating.[2] These violent remedies were the collective cornerstones of "Heroic Medicine," a type of treatment for disease that originated in Europe and found its way to the United States.[3] The aim of contemporary physicians was to rid the body of infections and illness by bleeding or by purging and flushing out the intestines, then inducing sweat to perspire out the rest of the toxins.

Bleeding

An excess of blood was blamed for many illnesses, including the fevers that arose from infectious diseases, headaches, and epilepsy. Bleeding was thought to reduce the inflammation that accompanied these diseases. An overabundance of blood was also blamed for "morbid excitement" and irritability in a patient.

Bleeding a patient was accomplished by cutting open a small vein and allowing blood to drain out. The cut was typically placed near the site of the pain or illness. For example, bleeding a vein under the tongue was used to cure a sore throat. Cutting was accomplished by using either a lancet (a sharp surgical knife, also called a fleam) or a scarificator, which was a metal box with a series of spring-loaded cutting blades.

Differential diagnosis to separate out specific illnesses was not necessarily considered to be important, and variations in treatment consisted primarily of when, where, how often, and how extensively bleeding should be performed.

How much blood to remove was problematic. Some enthusiastic doctors removed as much as a quart of blood every forty-eight hours. Typically, the sicker the patient, the more blood was drained out. Physicians sometimes judged the amount of blood to remove by gauging the way the patient responded. They watched for symptoms such as fluttering of the pulse, pale lips, a blue-gray tint around the eyes, a decreased awareness of pain, and lethargy that bordered on unconsciousness. Considering the amount of blood that was sometimes removed, these symptoms were certainly understandable.

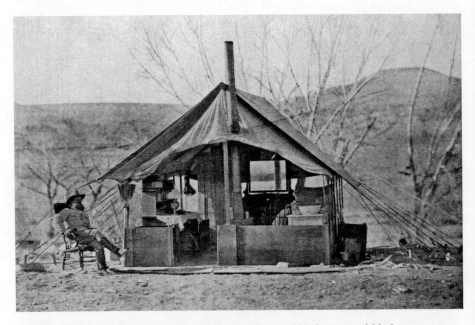

Army surgeons in the West believed that plenty of fresh air would help to restore health. This officer is essentially camping out in a tent at Fort Stanton, New Mexico. Established in 1855 to fight in the Indian Wars, Fort Stanton was converted to a federal tuberculosis hospital in 1899 (National Library of Medicine).

Benjamin Rush, one of the leading medical thinkers of his day and an eminent physician in Philadelphia (also a signer of the Declaration of Independence), is often considered to be the father of American medicine. He believed that up to four-fifths of the blood in the body should be bled in extreme cases. The problem was that doctors did not know at the time how much blood the body contained. Some thought that it held twelve quarts, not the six that it actually holds.

The use of bleeding as a cure started to lose its popularity during the middle decades of the 1800s, and by 1860 it had mostly fallen into disuse in the East. However, it was still a common form of treatment in the California gold fields in 1849, and some practitioners in the West continued bleeding patients well into the 1870s. As late as 1875, a paper on bleeding was presented at a meeting of the Rocky Mountain Medical Association. Bleeding was still used occasionally as late as the 1930s as a treatment for high blood pressure (hypertension).[4]

Purging

Bleeding was one of the two main foundations of Heroic Medicine. The other was purging the intestinal tract, a process that supposedly expelled the cause of the disease and rebalanced the humors. Cleansing the bowels was accomplished by using a series of medicines that consisted of laxatives, cathartics, and purgatives.[5]

The most popular medicine for purging was calomel (mercurous chloride), which was found in almost every home medicine chest and which was frequently prescribed by doctors. Another was jalap, which was derived from the plant *convolvulus jalapa*, and had an effect that was both dramatic and explosive.

The particular type of medicine used to accomplish purging for a specific disease or case depended on how violent and complete the results were supposed to be. Clysters (enemas) were also commonly used, either to achieve the same cleansing effect or if, for some reason, the oral route for purgative medicines was not possible.

The following illustrates the dogged lengths to which physicians went to cleanse the system. Before Lewis and Clark started their famous exploration of the West in 1803–06, they consulted physician Benjamin Rush in Philadelphia. His medical advice for disease included "gently opening the bowels by means of one, two, or more of the purging pills." The pills that Rush supplied were a purgative medicine that he had patented. He called them "Rush's Pills," or "bilious pills," but they were known more ominously by users as "Thunderclappers." Rush was convinced that they should be used for all ailments. They were made from a combination of calomel and jalap, and as historian Stephen Ambrose commented, "Each drug was a purgative of explosive power."[6] The medical supplies that Rush advised Lewis and Clark take with them included a clyster syringe for enemas, but the men reportedly preferred to take Rush's pills. Obviously expecting bad times, the expedition took an amazing 600 of Rush's Thunderclappers with them.

In spite of the expedition's magnificent pharmacopoeia, when Lewis and Clark reached Oregon, most of the men were ill with dysentery, diarrhea, and vomiting. Clark responded valiantly by administering Rush's pills indiscriminately. This was probably not a good idea, and he noted, "Several men So unwell that they were Compelled to lie on the Side of the road for Some time."[7] Never one to give up, Clark administered more of Rush's pills. The next day, when he found that Lewis was still sick, Clark gave him some laxative salts, tartar emetic, and jalap. It took Lewis about a week to recover.

Forty years later, Francis Parkman described the treatment of a companion who was struck down on the prairie in 1846 with what he called "brain fever." At Bent's Fort on the Arkansas River in today's Colorado, the ailing man was placed in the fort's sick chamber — a little mud room — with another ill man, and both were wrapped in a buffalo robe. One man died. Parkman described the treatment: "The assistant-surgeon's deputy visited them once a day and brought them each a huge dose of calomel, the only medicine, according to his surviving victim, with which he was acquainted."[8]

Just as the loss of blood achieved by bleeding usually calmed the patient due to exhaustion, so did violent purging of the bowels. Therefore, to some extent, blood-letting and purging did suppress symptoms—though obviously not the causes of the disease.

Vomiting

Another method for supposedly expelling disease-causing humors (this time from the *other* end of the internal tract) was to use an emetic drug to induce violent vomiting. Popular medicines to achieve this were ipecac, made from the dried roots of a South American plant, and tartar emetic, which was composed of antimony and potassium tartarate.

Sweating and Blistering

Used in conjunction with bleeding, purging, and vomiting, two popular supplemental treatments used in Heroic Medicine were sweating and blistering. The theory was that sweating and blistering were alternative treatments to draw bad humors out of the body by forcing them to escape through the skin.

The most popular medicine to induce sweating, called a sudorific, was

Dover's Powder, which was a mixture of opium, ipecac, and lactose. Other medicines used were ipecac by itself, tartar emetic, and potassium nitrate.

Blistering was accomplished by applying various irritating chemical agents to the skin that caused large blisters to appear. The theory was that this procedure drew poisonous products to the surface of the skin and collected them in the form of large blisters, which sucked the "bad" humors from the body.

By the 1850s, these "heroic" cures were starting to fall into disfavor among the leading medical authorities in the East. In the West, however, these "cures" endured for several more decades. Many of the medical practices in the Midwest from the period 1840 to 1870 were still being practiced in the Old West up to the end of the century. By the close of the nineteenth century, Heroic Medicine, however, along with many of its medications, had been discarded.

Foul Miasmas and Heroic Cures

By the middle of the nineteenth century, medicine in the Old West had not advanced much beyond the humoral theories of the ancient Greeks, a situation that resulted in an inability to effectively prevent or treat illness. Because the true causes of infectious diseases—bacteria and viruses—were not discovered until the late 1800s, many illnesses were blamed on "miasmas." A miasma was the foul, smelly vapor that arose from swamps, and similarly pervaded sewers and rotting food in garbage piles. In the late 1700s, Benjamin Rush believed that the cause of malaria was putrid exhalations of decayed animal and vegetable matter. He recommended closing doors and windows of houses at dusk to protect the occupants from "night airs," and thus prevent sickness.

This view was carried on well into the nineteenth century. As one medical manual put it: "The deleterious effluvia arising from the decomposition of vegetable substances; from persons in a state of disease; from putrid animal substances; are among the remote, but not least exciting causes, of fever." The author should have thought about what he was writing, because he went on to say: "Daily experience confirms the fact that in the neighborhood of marshes, and all such places, where vegetable and animal putrefaction takes place to any extent, pestilential and other diseases of various grades and violence, prevail."[9] He had the answer — something coming from the swamps — but didn't see it. The true causes of disease — microorganisms — were not discovered for several more decades.

In the meantime, bad environments were considered to generate stenches and "bad air," which, in turn, resulted in disease. Diseases were generally considered to fall into two main categories: miasmatic diseases and non-miasmatic diseases. Miasmatic diseases included what were called intermittent, eruptive, and continued fevers.

Intermittent fevers were the result of diseases, such as malaria, that had a recurrent nature, during which symptoms would periodically flare up and then die down again. Eruptive fevers were characterized by skin eruptions and a rise in body temperature. Yellow fever was considered to be an eruptive fever because one symptom of the disease was a rash that broke out on the skin. Other examples of eruptive fevers were measles and smallpox. Continued fevers were also called "camp fevers" or "crowd poisoning." One disease classified as a continued fever was typhoid, another was salmonella (food poisoning). The standard "heroic" treatment for miasmatic fevers was bleeding or purging, or both, with perhaps some sweating and vomiting for eruptive fevers thrown in for good measure.

The second general category was non-miasmatic diseases, which included respiratory tract inflammations and infections, such as pneumonia. Attempts to cure these diseases included the application of hot plasters to the chest. In cases of severe respiratory problems, the patient was sometimes bled, the thinking being that by doing so the lungs wouldn't have to work as hard. In reality, of course, bleeding reduced the amount of red blood cells that were available to carry oxygen throughout the body, which meant that the lungs had to work even harder to compensate for the loss of blood.

The treatments prescribed for fever were hard on a patient who was already feeling ill and weak. The following is a typical example:

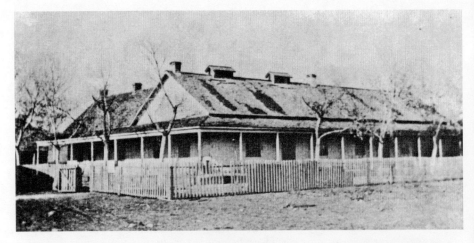

The post hospital at Fort Verde, Arizona, was a wooden structure that had ten beds. Supervised by a hospital matron, the hospital was used strictly as a convalescent ward and medicine dispensary (author's collection).

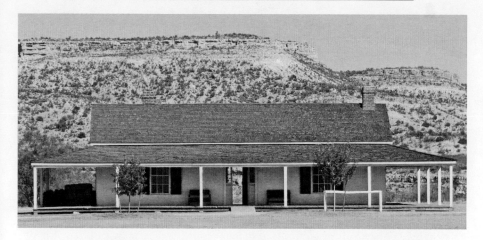

Surgery and treatment of the ill and wounded at Fort Verde took place in the doctor's quarters (author's collection).

> Give first suitable stimulants to raise the internal heat, as the alterative powders [a generalized non-specific tonic], cayenne pepper, vegetable elixir, &c. Then apply the vapor or steam bath ... until a brisk perspiration is produced; then give the stimulating injection ... and then emetic ... and repeat it until it operates thoroughly. Then when the patient is a little rested, apply the vapor bath again ... then give a moderate cathartic, merely sufficient to cause a slight action of the bowels. Then give the alterative powders, or other stimulants, once in two or three hours, to keep up the internal heat; and repeat the above course at intervals of from twelve to forty-eight hours, until relief in obtained.[10]

This must have been an approach of kill or cure.

Mental Illness

Mental illness was not generally understood, and treatment of those with mental conditions was primitive or non-existent. Benjamin Rush believed that mental illness was a result of too much blood in the brain. As a result, he advocated his favorite treatment, bloodletting. As with other diseases, the removal of large quantities of blood had a "calming" effect; thus Rush felt that he had developed a viable treatment. Under his medical blessing, this practice continued into the nineteenth century.

Others regarded mental illness as God's punishment for some evil deed that the person had committed, and the insane were typically hidden away out of the sight of mainstream society. Victorian moral reformers claimed that insanity was a result of immorality or some other sin. Though not understood at the time, in a perverted way this concept had some validity, because many of the inmates of mental asylums were those who had contracted syphilis, which had advanced to the point where the disease had destroyed much of their brain tissue.

Many hospitals would not accept the mentally ill, the senile, the clinically depressed, the retarded, and other victims of mental illness. Those with mental disorders were locked in prisons alongside criminals, in almshouses, or locked in the attic at home. Some considered the insane to be possessed by evil spirits, and these demons were often exorcised by violent means.[11] One supposed cure for insanity was to apply a blistering agent to the shaven head of a mentally ill person. Trephining, or drilling into the skull, to supposedly release disease-causing agents, was also used.

In the mid-nineteenth century many mentally ill individuals were chained in asylums or committed to local county jails because nobody knew what to do with them. By the 1880s, mental problems started to become recognized as an illness, and institutions to care for victims were slowly improved.

Two curious mental illnesses that were a product of the Victorian age have since disappeared. One was a disease of women called hysteria, the primary symptoms of which would now be considered to be a combination of paranoia and manic depression. The corresponding mental disease that was peculiar to Victorian men in the second half of the nineteenth century was neurasthenia, which was thought to be brought on by the stresses of contemporary modern life.

Hysteria

The name of this ethereal disorder was derived from *hustera*, the Greek name for the womb. Among other symptoms were headaches, fainting, insomnia, difficulty in breathing, unprovoked fits of laughter or crying, depression, and morbid, unfounded fears. The manifestation of these symptoms was considered to be composed of three related disorders: hysteria, chlorosis, and neurasthenia. The symptoms of all three (as they were then defined) were similar and overlapping. To add to the confusion, in an earlier historical context, hysteria was thought to be due to vapors from fermented menses; therefore, women suffering from hysterical attacks were said to be having "an attack of the vapors."

Ancient Greek and Egyptian medical theory blamed hysteria on the uterus, which they felt became inflamed or became somehow detached and wandered through the body looking for fulfillment. By the nineteenth century, physicians realized that the uterus was permanently attached in place by muscles and ligaments, but still continued to blame it for mental disorders in women. In view of this "enlightened" thinking, hysteria was theorized to be due to factors such as bad physical or moral education, living in a city, overindulgence in coffee and tea, and a bad constitution.

One description of hysteria was that it "is characterized by a grumbling noise in the bowels; a sense of suffocation as though a ball was ascending to the throat; stupor, insensibility, convulsions, laughing and crying without any visible cause; sleep interrupted by sighing and groaning, attended with flatulence and nervous symptoms. It is caused by affections of the womb, &c."[12]

Eventually, general medical agreement was that hysteria was probably caused by sexual deprivation, as it often affected young unmarried women, nuns, and widows. Where possible, marriage was the recommended course of action for a cure. Other treatments consisted of various spa therapies, such as using high-pressure jets of hot and cold water to buffet the body, and an extended course of treatment drinking mineral water. Flogging the patient with wet towels or sheets was a more vigorous spa treatment. As always, the old standby of purging emerged as a treatment, as it was thought to rid the body of putrifying waste that might be causing problems by accumulating in the lower abdomen around the sexual organs.

The term "chlorosis," often used interchangeably at the time with hysteria, was a disease of young women that was also thought to have a uterine origin. It was alternately called "greensickness" because the victim's complexion took on a greenish hue. At the time, the cause was variously attributed to anemia, anorexia, or hysteria. The treatment was the same as for hysteria, perhaps with some dietary iron added to spa water, which would have cured the anemia. The more modern meaning of chlorosis refers to a form of iron-deficiency anemia, particularly in young women. This type of chlorosis is not seen today because of modern nutrition.

Closely associated with hysteria in the male-oriented medical mind was pain during women's monthly periods, which was conjectured to be due to misguided personal and social habits of the individual. As an extension of this idea, Orson S. Fowler, a male social critic, contended in 1870 that pain that occurred during menstruation was due to "uterine congestion" brought on by excessive reading of romantic novels. Recommended treatment included avoidance of novels and any intellectual pursuits, and a daily dosing with tonics.

After 1895, when Drs. Josef Breuer and Sigmund Freud published *Studies in Hysteria*, the disease passed into the realm of psychoanalysis and eventually faded from the medical scene as a specific ailment.

Neurasthenia

Neurasthenia was the corresponding mental disease that appeared in Victorian men. Among other symptoms that must have been confusing to the sufferer and diagnostician, it was said to be characterized by a series of odd and vague symptoms that included an extreme sensitivity to weather changes, tenderness in the teeth, excessive sensitivity to being tickled, itching, hot flashes, sweating hands, writer's cramp, and yawning. The disease did not appear in working men, such as farmers, cowboys, or miners, but was only diagnosed in men with jobs that required them to use mental exertion. Neurasthenia was claimed to strike men such as doctors, lawyers, and inventors—all of whom were individuals who worked with their brains. It was felt to be linked to increased intellectual development in the Victorian American male, and was accepted as a sign of mental superiority. Among the causes, according to Dr. George Beard, in an 1881 book entitled *American Nervousness: Its Causes and Consequences*, were "sexual excesses, the abuse of stimulants and narcotics, and sudden retirement from business." Treatments were similar to those for hysteria.

One form of treatment for neurasthenia, after the development of electrotherapy devices, was electrical stimulation that used various electrodes applied either to the skin or inserted into various body openings. Other treatments used various elixirs, tonics, and patent medicines. One device that was widely advertised to offer a cure was a form of electric hairbrush. Among the recommended cures were a series of mineral water treatments, which were also claimed at the same time to cure gout, anemia, paralysis, hysteria, laryngitis, flatulence, and liver problems.

Closely allied with neurasthenia and hysteria was "hypochondrial melancholy," a disease supposedly caused by an excess of the classical humor "black bile" that had accumulated in the lower abdomen. It was named after the *hypochondrium*, which is the medical term for that part of the abdomen on each side of the body below the ribs. Hypochondrial melancholy was also associated with privileged individuals and became a "disease" of intellectual superiority. The "cure" was a good purging to remove the excess bile. Over time, the meaning of the term changed, and "hypochondriasis" became applied to those who were affected by a morbid obsession with psychosomatic ailments.

After 1900, the diagnosis of neurasthenia was also applied to women, making hysteria, chlorosis, and neurasthenia three interchangeable and confusingly nebulous diseases. Reference sources on all three diseases are muddled and often contradictory, and the meanings of the terms have changed over time.[13]

Progress and Understanding

As the second half of the nineteenth century progressed, so did advances in medicine, as the true causes of many diseases were gradually discovered.

Some of the most important findings came from the significant advances in bacteriology that started to take place in the mid–1800s. Bacteriology, as a field of study, emerged in the 1830s, was the focus of major efforts in the 1840s and 1850s, and started to see significant results in the 1860s. In 1862, for example, French chemist Louis Pasteur established a link between microscopic organisms (microbes) and fermentation.

Between 1870 and 1905, French and German bacteriologists (notably Robert Koch in Germany) identified the organisms that were involved in many of the serious infectious diseases that were rampant in the Old West, such as cholera, typhoid, tuberculosis, pneumonia, diphtheria, tetanus, bubonic plague, gonorrhea, and syphilis. In 1876, for example, Robert Koch proved that a specific bacillus caused anthrax. Koch's discovery of the tuberculosis bacillus in 1882 led to treatments for the disease. It was not until after the turn of the twentieth century, however, that sanitary treatment of water and food, along with the control of insect vectors (particularly for mosquitoes), began to check the spread of diseases such as typhoid, cholera, yellow fever, and malaria. Death rates from these diseases dropped dramatically in the early 1900s as various measures to improve cleanliness were instituted.

Developments in measuring instruments that occurred during the second half of the nineteenth century allowed better understanding and diagnosis of diseases. By 1880, physicians were starting to routinely use pulse, temperature, and blood pressure as indicators of the state of a patient's health. An increase in the use and understanding of diagnostic techniques, such as taking a patient's temperature, helped in the differentiation and diagnosis of specific diseases. Progress in diagnosis was made with the simple recognition that fever was a symptom of a disease and not the disease itself.

Before a useful version of the clinical thermometer was developed, a physician obtained a crude indication of a patient's body temperature and suspected fever simply by touching the patient's skin. A thermometer that could be used in the mouth had been developed in the 1600s by Santorio Santorio, but it was not until the mid–1800s that physicians started to use the thermometer as a diagnostic tool. Part of this reluctance was due to a lack of understanding of the meaning of abnormal body temperature, and part was due to limitations in the measuring device.

Early versions of the clinical thermometer had to be kept in contact with a patient's armpit for up to twenty minutes to achieve a stable and accurate reading of body temperature, and the device did not hold the measurement, but had to be read while it was still in contact with the patient. Some clinical thermometers were fully twelve inches long, which made them unwieldy to carry in a doctor's bag and use on the patient. Progress in technology gradually overcame these limitations, resulting in the development of a version similar to the modern clinical thermometer in 1867 by Thomas Clifford All-butt in England.

Clinical thermometers were slow to be adopted by rural doctors in the Old West. The designs were so fragile that thermometers often broke while being carried around in the doctor's saddlebags. Instead, the frontier doctor became expert at feeling for fever by touch.

The stethoscope, another major diagnostic advance, was invented in 1816 by French physician René Théophile Hyacinthe Laënnec, but, like the thermometer, the device did not receive widespread use in the Old West until late in the nineteenth century. Laënnec conceived the idea for a stethoscope when he was called to examine an overweight young woman who was having chest pains. In this case, the woman's excessive weight did not allow the use of percussion (tapping the chest and listening for the resulting sounds) because her body fat muffled the sounds. Before the invention of the stethoscope, when a doctor wanted to listen specifically for irregular heart sounds, he put his ear on the patient's chest. Laënnec was embarrassed to put his ear directly on the young woman's ample bosom because he felt that this would be an affront to her modesty. After thinking for a while about how to solve the problem, a flash of inspiration gave him the idea of using a rolled-up bundle of papers as an extended listening tube.

The concept worked so well that Laënnec later experimented with different designs to improve on the roll of paper. He finally came up with a hollow, resonant tube, about nine inches long and an inch-and-a-half in diameter, made from wood. The physician could place one end of the tube to his ear and the other to the patient's chest, and was thus able to hear heartbeats clearly. A binaural version of the stethoscope, for use with both ears, with ivory earpieces and flexible rubber tubing was developed in 1852 by physician George Cammann. As doctors learned to understand the meaning of different chest and abdominal sounds, the stethoscope gained additional use as an instrument for detecting noises that could be used to diagnose internal disorders.

CHAPTER TWO

Doctors and Healers

Becoming a Doctor

Part of the problem with medical care in the early West was a shortage of doctors. At the time the frontier was pushing west towards California, there were no medical schools west of the Mississippi. Doctors with medical degrees from institutions of higher learning in the East were few, and even then the quality of formal education received by doctors varied tremendously.

The choices for becoming a doctor in the mid–1800s were three. The preferred method was to attend medical school in Europe. The second choice was to attend one of the few medical schools in the United States. The third, which was the commonest and the traditional pathway to becoming a doctor at mid-century, was to serve for several years as an apprentice to a practicing physician.

Those individuals who had plenty of money and wanted the best education went to medical school on the European Continent. The Royal College of Physicians in Edinburgh, Scotland, for example, was considered to be a world center for medical education. Other important medical schools were in Paris, London, and Leyden, Germany. Medical students attended lectures for four years, receiving laboratory training and clinical experience during their studies. They then returned to the United States to practice. Most, however, chose to set up their practices in the cities of the East, where they found they could have the best facilities and attract the most lucrative patients. There was no incentive for these doctors to go to the frontier.

One of the alternatives to becoming a doctor was to attend one of the few medical schools that were available in the United States for those with enough money to afford them. The University of Pennsylvania, in Philadelphia, had been educating doctors since 1762. Harvard, Yale, and Princeton were established centers of learning. Would-be doctors attended a series of lectures, passed an examination, and could be licensed to practice medicine in as little as a year. In 1830 there were twenty-two medical schools in the

United States. By 1850 there were forty-two, and by 1861 the number had grown to eighty-seven.

Attending medical school was not inexpensive, but help might come from unexpected sources. Etta Murphy, known affectionately as "Spuds," owned a bordello named Murphy's Resort Saloon in Pueblo, Colorado. She helped put her brother through medical school with money that she earned from her whorehouse.

The course of instruction in these early medical schools typically consisted of three to five months of formal lectures, then apprenticeship to a practicing physician for the rest of the year to complete the practical part of the education. This same course of study might be repeated by students the next year to give them two years of experience.

The teachers at these early medical schools were also practicing physicians. The coursework consisted mostly of a series of pedantic lectures, which might be arbitrarily canceled if the doctor who was teaching at the time had to see one of his patients. Another disadvantage was that there was little or no practical hands-on laboratory work. Most American medical schools did not have laboratories, certainly not anatomy laboratories, because there was a lack of bodies for dissection. Religious beliefs led most people to object to anyone — even doctors and medical students—cutting up dead bodies. Most doctors had to learn surgical techniques by practicing on live patients. After becoming a doctor, many did not perform surgery very often unless it was a last resort because they had not received the training to properly perform it.

Medical research was limited to observing, while the teacher lectured on what he considered to be a few interesting or unusual cases. Another severe limitation was that there were few medical libraries to support any learning. Diagnostic equipment might also be non-existent or in short supply. During the Civil War, for example, Harvard Medical School did not have a stethoscope or a microscope. This may, however, be an unfair criticism, as medical students usually purchased their own stethoscopes rather than using one from the school.

The third method of becoming a doctor in the latter part of the nineteenth century was via the apprentice system, a method that dated from the 1700s.[1] Apprentices learned anatomy, surgery, and the compounding of medicines by practice on the job. They joined a doctor in daily care of patients, dressing wounds, performing bloodletting and minor surgery, and pulling teeth. In exchange for learning, apprentices might also have to clean the doctor's office, run his errands, and take care of his horses. Would-be doctors performed this apprenticeship for between two and six years, then received a certificate of proficiency that allowed them to start their own practice.

This method of training was common well into the late 1800s. A study of eighty-nine doctors in Clear Creek County, Colorado, for example, who practiced between 1865 and 1895, estimated that one-third had not attended formal medical school.[2] In 1883, one physician in the West, Dr. Josiah Hall, estimated that 85 percent of doctors were still being trained by another doctor. In 1885 only half of the doctors in Butte, Montana, had been trained at recognized medical schools.

At the time that the Civil War started in 1861, there were no common standards for earning an MD degree, and the result was an uneven quality of doctors. In the 1870s even as prestigious an institution as the Harvard Medical School did not give written examinations because many of the students were not able to write well enough. It was not until the end of the nineteenth century that medical schools such as Johns Hopkins came into existence and required a college degree for entrants.

There were few licensing laws and regulations; therefore, many individuals who practiced were unqualified or had minimal background and training. In the rural West this may have accounted for over a quarter of the doctors. In the 1849–50 gold rush days of California, one observer speculated that probably only about thirty had genuine credentials out of the 200 in San Francisco who called themselves doctor.

By 1880 there were one hundred medical schools in the United States, and by the late 1800s the system of training under an experienced physician was gradually replaced by a formal education. Change was slow, however. Even in the 1870s it was possible to purchase a diploma through the mail, and by 1879 only seven out of the thirty-eight states in the Union had effective licensing laws. Medical licensing did not become prevalent until the 1890s.

The Doctor as Healer

Physicians on the Western frontier were generalists. They had to perform surgery, deliver a baby, diagnose and treat illnesses, and perhaps occasionally pull a tooth. Babies were delivered at home, and surgery to treat accidents was often performed on the patient's kitchen table. As a result, doctors in rural areas spent long hours on the road between cases. Traveling thirty miles by horse and buggy to a distant ranch to treat a sick patient or deliver a baby was not unusual. A few doctors in large cities limited themselves to specific diseases and ailments, but the age of the specialist did not really start until the early 1900s.

Veterinarians were even scarcer in the Old West than doctors. A doctor might be asked to treat a family cow or a horse, if no veterinarian was available, because a healthy horse was important to a farmer or rancher. Many doctors also owned drugstores and served as pharmacists.

Doctors made house calls, either by wagon or horse and buggy, or they rode a horse, with their surgical kit and drugs stowed in saddlebags behind them. A team of horses pulling a buckboard could go about seven or eight miles an hour in good weather on a good road. Thus, a forty-mile trip to an outlying ranch could take four or five hours, one way, to complete. In poor weather or on muddy roads, progress might be reduced to only three miles per hour. It was not unusual for a doctor to spend fourteen hours on the round trip to visit a single patient.

The doctor's equipment on these field visits consisted of a black bag filled mostly with knives, probes, saws, obstetrical instruments, forceps, clamps, needles, and sutures.[3] One side of the saddle bags carried stoppered glass medicine bottles so that the doctor could measure out the appropriate drugs during his visit. Common medicines carried in saddlebags were jalap, calomel, quinine, and laudanum.

Doctors looked at skin color, and observed the patient for swelling or inflammation. Physical examination was limited, because touching the patient's body, particularly a woman's, was considered to be indelicate. A doctor might feel the pulse, look at the tongue, listen for coughs or breathing difficulties, and note any unusual odors. Patients dying from tuberculosis, for example, had offensive breath due to the progression of decay in their lungs. Physician Arthur Hertzler described what many doctors did when called to a sick patient: "He greeted the patient with a grave look and a pleasant joke. He felt the pulse and inspected the tongue, and asked where it hurt. This done, he was ready to deliver an opinion and prescribe his pet remedy."[4]

Many diagnoses were obvious, such as a sore throat, asthma, or rheumatism. Injuries were sewn up and broken bones were splinted with a board from the barnyard. In cases of severe illness, a doctor might call on a patient several times a day, and frequently sit with a dying patient until the end.

Surgery was often performed on the kitchen table. Similar to battlefield surgery, the correct technique was to operate fast to prevent exposure of tissues to bacteria in the air. Arthur Hertzler mentioned that one time he had operated outside under an apple tree.

By the end of the century, closer scrutiny of the patient was more common and included feeling the pulse, measuring the blood pressure, taking the temperature, and conducting a thorough physical examination. The examination followed a standardized ritual. It opened with some conversation to set the patient and the family at ease, followed by the doctor solemnly checking the pulse, feeling the forehead and face for fever, pressing the abdomen for tender areas or enlarged organs, and listening to the heart and lungs with a stethoscope. Then, after a short, suitable period of meditation came the diagnosis. The ritual was completed by dispensing a suitable medicine, and the doctor was back on his horse or in his buggy and on to the next patient.

Telephones, of course, were not available to summon a doctor in cases of illness or emergency. Telephones did not appear in doctors' offices in Colorado, for example, until 1879. Then they were available only in the big cities, such as Denver.

Likewise, the doctor could not jump into a car to rush to attend to a patient. Automobiles did not appear in the West until about 1890. Even then, if the dirt road to an isolated house call was rough and rutted, or the road was snow-packed and icy, it was often easier and more reliable for the doctor to use a horse.

The vast open spaces of the West meant that there might be serious delays in summoning medical help in the case of serious illness or an accident. A family member or ranch hand might have to ride forty or fifty miles to the nearest town to find a doctor, and then both would have to ride the same distance back again. In some instances it could be several days before the doctor arrived. Mud, snow, rain, and cold made many of these trips less than pleasant. In winter, ice, snow, or a river swollen by spring floods turned the journey into an ordeal.

Patients expected doctors to achieve cures that might be impossible, but, by the same token, doctors sometimes promised more than they could deliver. One factor that often played a part in the outcome of treatment was that victims of disease or an accident did not go to the doctor until it was too late for a cure. In all fairness, many diseases had insidious beginnings and did not show any distressing symptoms until the disease was well-advanced. In such cases, any minor symptoms were often ignored until too late.

Luckily, many diseases were self-limiting; that is to say that, given enough time and rest, the body cured itself. All the doctor had to do in these cases was to provide supportive care or some placebo medicine until the patient recovered by himself.

Treatment was sometimes delayed either because of the distance to reach the doctor's office or the cost of a visit to the doctor. Though the doctor's fee might be only five dollars for a home visit, a fee of a dollar a mile might be added on for travel—perhaps double that at night or in bad weather. Poor people couldn't afford to see a doctor, especially in rural areas where cash was short. As a result, doctors were often sent for as a last resort, but by then it might be too late. In many cases, patients either got better by themselves or didn't and died.

Any failure to achieve a satisfactory cure, whether the fault lay with the doctor or the patient, resulted in a low level of confidence in doctors. Much of the deep-rooted skepticism of doctors in the Old West was caused by their limited success in curing illnesses. The blame should not be placed wholly on the doctor, however, because most illnesses were the result of infection or disease agents whose causes were unknown at the time. Also, ill people were reluctant to go to the doctor, which resulted in a high rate of mortality. The high death rate, in turn, made sick people more reluctant to visit the doctor, which resulted in a vicious circle that delayed treatment.

Doctors spent much of their time dealing with fevers caused by bacterial invasions. Not much could be done for the patient but to provide good cheer and supportive care. If positive action was called for, the treatment might be to perform bloodletting or purging the bowels to try to drive out the infectious agents.

The Doctor's Office

The offices of many of the first doctors in the West were located in tents and log cabins. In small communities the office might be in a hotel room or in the back of a store. Often the patient was treated in a room at the back of the doctor's home. Eventually, as towns became established and grew larger, doctors moved their offices into bank buildings and other professional office buildings, alongside lawyers and accountants.

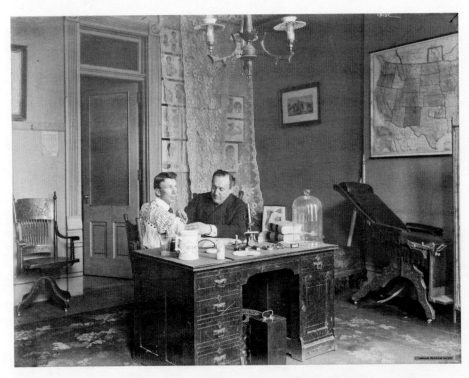

Typical doctor's office in Denver, Colorado, at the turn of the century, with the doctor (thought to be Dr. L.F. Preston) administering an injection to a patient (copyright, Colorado Historical Society; Buckwalter Collection, Scan #20031405).

A doctor's office in the Old West was typically furnished with a wooden desk, a bookcase full of impressive-looking medical reference books, and a cabinet for storing and displaying medical instruments. A reclining chair or padded leather table in the middle of the office was used for examinations and minor surgery. Shelves held bottles of chemicals for dispensing medicines or salves. The doctor himself was typically dressed in the standard physician's uniform of the day, which consisted of a black Prince Albert coat and a top hat.

The doctor dispensed medicine while the patient was in the office or the doctor was in the patient's home. Dispensing drugs by physicians was a necessary addition to diagnosis, because there was often no practical way for a patient in a small town, or one who lived on a remote ranch, to obtain necessary medicines. There were few prepared medicines, so doctors typically purchased chemicals in bulk, and compounded and dispensed them as required for individual use. Doctors making house calls in remote areas usually carried folding scales and druggist's equipment so that they could measure out the required medications before they left the patient.

For all this effort, the pay for a doctor was not particularly good. The

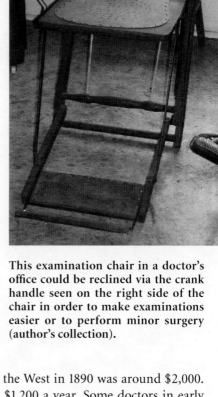

This examination chair in a doctor's office could be reclined via the crank handle seen on the right side of the chair in order to make examinations easier or to perform minor surgery (author's collection).

average annual income for a doctor in the West in 1890 was around $2,000. In the smaller towns it was as little as $1,200 a year. Some doctors in early mining camps or small rural Western towns found it difficult to make ends meet. A rural doctor might get as little as fifty cents for an office visit. Many doctors were paid in chickens, eggs, bacon, or whatever crops a rancher or farmer raised. As a result, few doctors wanted to move out West.

The charge for an office exam was typically between $5 and $10. For a

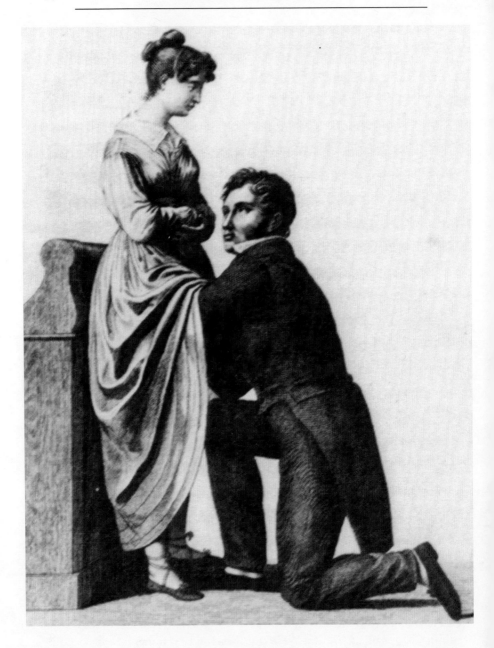

Examination of female patients was often difficult for the doctor, who had to feel under or through layers of clothing in order to preserve the patient's modesty (author's collection).

simple delivery, $25; for a complex delivery, $50 to $200. Treatment of gonorrhea was between $25 and $30, and for syphilis was $40 to $100. The prices that doctors charged for their services stayed relatively stable from the 1860s to the turn of the century.[5]

Part of the financial problem might be that unpaid bills went overdue, and the doctor couldn't collect enough cash to make his own living. Ranch owners often sold crops or cattle only once or twice a year and in between had no ready cash. In these instances, much of the doctor's earnings were in trade. Even if a doctor did not want to barter, but wanted cash, he often had to settle for a side of beef or a few chickens for the stew pot in order to survive.

As a result of these difficult conditions, medicine was not always a full-time job in small towns. Doctors also farmed, mined, raised cattle, sold real estate, and dabbled in banking on the side. Some doctors also had additional careers as businessmen, real estate developers, loan officers, drug store owners, hotel owners, or newspaper reporters. Doctors were involved in freighting, running boardinghouses, bartending, or prospecting for gold and silver.

There might also be hefty competition for patients. In 1875, Virginia City, Nevada, had forty-seven doctors and dentists for a census figure of a little over 10,000 adults. Leadville in 1880 had fifty-eight physicians to serve an estimated population of 15,000. In 1897, Cripple Creek, Colorado, had fifty-five doctors and ten dentists for a population of 30,000. In 1901, Denver had one doctor for every 300 residents. As a result, there was often not enough work to go around.

In 1889, Illinois had an estimated 1,500 to 2,000 doctors, considerably more than were needed to provide medical services. As a result of this glut, many did not earn a comfortable livelihood. On the other hand, in some very remote areas of the West there might not be enough doctors to serve those who needed medical care. The 1870 census of the Arizona Territory listed twenty-two civilian physicians and eleven army surgeons for the entire territory.

Treating women in the last half of the nineteenth century created some specialized problems for physicians. Victorian modesty did not permit nakedness, so doctors often had to examine female patients through their many layers of clothing, or have the patient point to a specific area of a picture or a doll to indicate where the source of the malady might be. In a similar fashion, if a doctor were present at childbirth, he might have to assist in the delivery by feel, under a blanket or sheet, in order to preserve the expectant mother's modesty. Childbirth usually took place at home, rather than in a hospital, and was attended by female midwives. When female physicians became more common later in the century, women often preferred to go to them, as they felt that another woman would be more sympathetic to women's unique medical problems, particularly issues such as menstrual difficulties or matters related to sex.

Women Physicians

There were few women physicians in the mid-to-late 1800s. Estimates are that fewer than sixty practiced in the Old West. The first woman physician in the United States, Elizabeth Blackwell, did not graduate from an American medical school, the Geneva College of Medicine in Geneva, New York, until 1849.

The primary reason for this imbalance was the contemporary attitude that existed towards women in the mid-to-late 1800s, which relegated them to a lower status than men. Victorian society encouraged male dominance, and women were considered to be inferior to men, both mentally and physically. As a result, women trying to become doctors faced resentment and hostility from male students and faculty. As late as 1895 the *Pacific Medical Journal* stated its opinion that "obviously there are many vocations in life which women cannot follow.... One of those directions is medicine."[6]

While attending medical school, it was felt to be indelicate for a woman to listen to a discussion of medical subjects in the presence of men. Women who did so were considered to be immodest for seeking to learn what were considered to be the "disgusting duties" that were associated with healing the human body. In any case, early Victorian medical opinion was that women who sought to educate themselves would develop oversized brains, a weak digestion, and constipated bowels. One physician was certain that if women studied too much their reproductive organs would shrivel and that they would grow beards like men.

One irascible doctor is said to have told a female medical student that women should not study medicine, but if they did, they should have their ovaries removed. With great presence of mind, she replied that this would be fine, but then men studying to be doctors should have their testicles removed.

Women doctors had to be self-sufficient to survive under these conditions and could not be intimidated easily. When Louise Black was working as a doctor at the Clark Mineral Springs Hospital in Pueblo, Colorado, she was accosted by a man as she was crossing a bridge that went over the neighboring railroad yards. She fought back and managed to throw him over the side of the bridge. She made her escape and didn't wait to learn the extent of his injuries.

If a woman succeeded in becoming a doctor, she might find that she was ostracized by male physicians and excluded from using hospitals. Practices for women physicians were mostly limited to women and children. Some men did not trust female physicians because most did not believe in prescribing whiskey as a cure-all.

Women patients often preferred female physicians because they could talk about female complaints to an understanding ear. They also preferred women doctors for reasons of modesty, particularly for physical examinations, and also when discussing the venereal diseases that were rampant in the latter half of the nineteenth century. By the same token, some women felt that male doctors were more capable than women doctors and preferred to seek out a man for treatment.

Change was gradual and slow, but by the end of the nineteenth century, approximately one-quarter of medical students were women. As a nod to women's modesty, male and female students were usually separated during dissection classes.

Hospitals

The first hospital in the United States was founded in Philadelphia in 1752 at the urging of Benjamin Franklin. Early hospitals were essentially almshouses or charity institutions. They were "poor houses" used to institutionalize the poor, orphans, and criminals. These primitive "hospitals" offered minimal medical care, with the idea that, in this way, the poor would not become dependent on government assistance.

The nature of medical practice in the early days of the Old West was such that there was not much need for a hospital. Treatment took place in the doctor's office. Childbirth usually took place at home, with midwives in attendance rather than a doctor. Most surgical operations were conducted in the home either because of a lack of hospitals or a fear of contracting disease due to the close quarters and proximity to other sick people.

Infected people were often taken to "hospitals," which were, in reality, pesthouses used in attempts to control epidemics. The intent was to protect the public from dread diseases by isolating contagious cases in these institutions, rather than to treat and cure patients. As a result, hospitals were viewed as a place to die instead of one in which to be cured. In Colorado Springs, Colorado, for example, the "county hospital" was a pesthouse for isolating communicable diseases. It was located about two miles outside the small town to prevent transmission of disease to the other residents. A small, separate cemetery nearby was used to bury the victims of smallpox and similar communicable diseases who died in the hospital.

Early hospitals were lit by kerosene lamps, heated with coal stoves, and had no indoor plumbing. Rural hospitals were worse than urban ones. Patients in these "hospitals" often contracted another disease while they were there. There were no efforts to separate or quarantine sick patients. A woman in labor, for example, might be placed in a bed next to a typhoid patient. Small wonder that the death toll in hospital wards could be as high as 40 percent. Many patients, however, survived these primitive conditions and dreadful diseases. About 70 percent of those with typhoid fever eventually recovered.

Hospitals were not common in the Old West until the 1890s. Before that time, the only hospitals might be army hospitals. Fort Garland, a military installation established in Colorado in 1858, had a hospital with twelve beds, a dispensary, a kitchen, and a dining room. Toilet facilities were primitive, consisting of a pit toilet located outside the hospital building.

Fort Union, in New Mexico, had a hospital that was considered to be one of the best in the West. The fort was once the largest military installation on the frontier, acting as the supply depot and headquarters for the Military Department of New Mexico. The hospital, which had thirty-six beds and a capacity of about sixty patients, was housed in a large, white, clapboard building that was staffed by two surgeons and eight support personnel.

Fort Laramie, in Wyoming, had a twelve-bed hospital that was built in

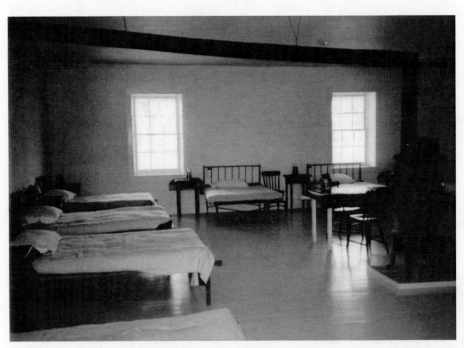

The post hospital at Fort Larned, Kansas, was a cheery place. The walls were white, and the floor was a bright yellow for cleanliness and to provide a cheerful atmosphere (courtesy Sylvia Agnew).

1873. Ironically, it was built on the site of the previous cemetery used by an earlier version of the fort. The hospital building was located at a distance from the main part of the fort, near the cavalry stables, with the idea that communicable diseases would be isolated there from the main body of soldiers.

Some of the first civilian "hospitals" in the Old West were simply rented rooms in a private house or a hotel, with untrained individuals hired to provide rudimentary nursing care to the sick. Doc Holliday, for example, spent the last days of his final illness in the Hotel Glenwood in Glenwood Springs, Colorado.

Hospitals were slow to be established in mining camps, both because of the cost and the uncertainty of the camp's future. If the mining strike played out, everyone moved quickly to the next strike. Catholic organizations eventually founded hospitals to care for those who could not afford to pay.

Mining companies and railroads often established their own hospitals to care for employees who were injured on the job. For example, in 1885 the Copper Queen mining company founded a hospital with sixteen beds in Bisbee, Arizona. The mining company ran the hospital for twenty years, until it was replaced by the fifty-bed Calumet and Arizona Hospital. In mining districts like these, hospitals were often supported by contracts with local mining companies. Unlike today's company-sponsored health insurance plans, the cost was paid by the miner. A typical fee was one dollar per month from each miner.

St. Vincent's Hospital in the silver-mining town of Leadville, Colorado, was built in 1879, and had twelve private rooms and forty beds. In 1895 a new operating theater was added. Cripple Creek, Colorado, founded in response to rich gold finds in 1891, built a small hospital in 1894.

Ouray, Colorado, built the small two-story Miner's Hospital in 1887, which first operated under the Sisters of Mercy and then as a mining hospital until 1957, when it became the town clinic. The hospital was closed in 1964 because it did not have an elevator, which was required by Colorado law. Ten patient rooms and a simple operating suite were on the second floor. The basement housed the kitchen and patient dining room, which had a large table in the middle of the room for communal meals. The room remained virtually unchanged over the years of the hospital's existence.

Not all hospitals were necessarily shining examples of medical care. An 1870 report described the post hospital at Camp Lowell (later Fort Lowell) in Arizona as an old adobe building on the main street of town, located too close to irrigated fields and the nearby river. Because of its location, the fort was plagued with malaria during the first years of its operation due to mosquitoes that were breeding in the river. In addition, the hospital was criticized for having a leaky roof that allowed rainwater to run down the interior walls, for its worn-out floors, and for having a series of covered-up privies under the floor of the building. Because of all these issues, the building was found to be unfit for use and was moved and rebuilt in 1873.

As advances in medical treatment took place, hospitals came to be seen more as places to tend the sick rather than merely places to isolate those with infectious diseases. By the 1890s, more hospitals were being built and current ones upgraded. By 1900, there were approximately 4,000 hospitals in the United States.

After major plagues of smallpox, diphtheria, and tuberculosis were brought under control in the early 1900s, hospitals were used for recovery from disease, and childbirth and surgery. The benefits of using a hospital came full circle. As patients submitted to surgery in hospitals earlier in their illnesses, the mortality rate decreased, thus making patients less afraid of hospitals and more likely to go there for surgery. Along with this change, the practice of medicine changed the location of family medical care from the home to the doctor's office, then to clinics and the outpatient department of a hospital.

Medical Care in the Military

The best place for medical care in the Old West was at an army post. The physician there was either a military surgeon or a contract surgeon. Military surgeons were commissioned army officers and were required to have a formal education at a recognized medical school. Contract surgeons were civilians hired when there was a shortage of army doctors. They remained civilians. They had no military rank and did not wear army uniforms. Contract physicians often had been trained under the apprentice system and might not have the qualifications and experience in treating battle wounds as their military counterparts.

Surgeons and assistant surgeons were assigned by the Medical Corps. In 1869 there were 161 commissioned medical officers for 32,698 troops at 239 posts. The authorized strength was for 222 medical officers. During the early 1870s, 175 contract surgeons were added to try and make up the shortage, but in 1874 Congress limited the number to a total of seventy-five. Army doctors were well paid compared to rank-and-file soldiers. An assistant surgeon earned $125 a month in the 1870s; a surgeon typically earned $215.

Each army regiment had a surgeon and assistant surgeon or contract physician on staff, and had either a sick bay or, at the larger posts, a hospital. The army originally thought that any good civilian physician could act as a military surgeon during the Indian Wars of the latter half of the nineteenth century. However, the practicalities of the frontier quickly showed that this was not true. For one thing, civilian doctors usually didn't know much about military matters and often did not take well to the military chain of command. Following military orders from superior officers in medical matters was seen as meddling in the doctor's area of medical expertise and responsibility. Such commands were often ignored. Secondly, treating the wounds of battle and amputating wounded extremities was very different than treating sore throats and stomach complaints in civilians. If contract doctors did not take to the military life and discipline, they sometimes just walked out without warning.

Army hospitals were intended primarily to serve the military staff and their families, along with friendly Indians and civilian employees at the post. In remote areas of the West, however, the doctors and army hospitals often treated local homesteaders and ailing travelers as well. Medical services for soldiers and their families was free. Civilians had to pay for their care, a typical amount being fifty cents per day. Military surgeons and ambulances also accompanied troops into the field to care for the sick and wounded.

Poor diet and a lack of proper sanitation often resulted in widespread disease at army posts and in the field. Soldiers commonly suffered from typhoid, typhus, smallpox, dysentery, and scurvy. This was not specific to the Old West. During the Civil War, the Union Army lost twice the number of men to disease than it did to injuries from battle.[7]

The post surgeon was assisted by hospital stewards who formed part of the permanent medical staff. They ranked above first sergeants but below commissioned officers. Depending on their rank and time in service, they were paid from twenty to thirty dollars a month at a time when ordinary enlisted men made thirteen dollars a month. Stewards assisted the surgeon with compounding and administering medicines, performed minor treatments, and were responsible for keeping the hospitals clean. Surgeons and hospital stewards were assisted by enlisted men who were assigned as nurses and helpers for a period of special duty. This duty was not popular among the enlisted men, as they were the ones who performed the unpleasant duties, such as bathing the sick, cleaning and dressing suppurating wounds, and emptying bedpans.

In addition to his other duties, the post surgeon was in charge of sanitation and general health at the fort. This included tasks such as making sure that the water supply was adequate and clean, the latrines were kept in sanitary order, and that garbage was properly disposed of.

Military surgeons also served as scientific officers, recording weather data and daily temperatures, along with the amount of rainfall and its effect on soil conditions. Some medical officers took a great interest in the natural sciences, collecting and writing about what they saw during tours of duty in the West. Elliot Coues, for example, was an assistant surgeon who also became an expert on arrow wounds while stationed at Fort Whipple in Arizona. As well as performing his regular medical duties, he found time to publish several important reference works on birds and mammals. Similarly, post surgeon Edward Vollum at Fort Belknap in Texas, and John Head at Fort Ripley in Minnesota, collected specimens that enhanced the scientific collections of the Smithsonian Institute in Washington, D.C. Edgar Mearns, who was stationed as an army doctor at Fort Verde, Arizona, from 1884 to 1888, was a noted naturalist who explored many of the prehistoric ruins in the area in his spare time.

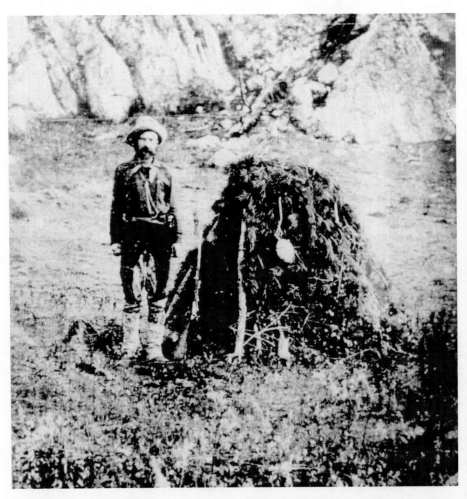

Army doctors often had to make do in the field. This ragged-looking individual is actually respected surgeon Valentine T. McGillycuddy, who accompanied General Crook's 1876 expedition to the Black Hills of South Dakota (National Archives).

During or after a major battle during the Indian Wars, army surgeons were responsible for setting up field hospitals, usually away from the main area of fighting. Such a "hospital" might be only a canvas wall tent, typically fourteen feet square, with four tall, vertical sides so that the surgeons and his support staff could stand and work in an upright position. A field hospital might house from six to twenty patients, depending on the size of the tent and the expedition.

If circumstances were otherwise, however, an army surgeon might have to make do as best he could. At the Battle of the Little Bighorn, where Lt. Col. George Armstrong Custer met his fate, Dr. Henry Porter was trapped on top of Reno Hill with Maj. Marcus Reno, Capt. Frederick Benteen, and their men. Porter had to improvise his "field hospital" in a simple depression in the ground, where he treated over fifty men who were wounded by gunshots and arrows.

Ambulances

The army was responsible for the introduction of ambulances as specialized vehicles for transport of the ill and wounded. Prior to the Civil War, the

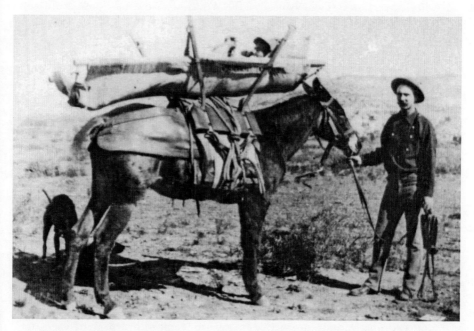

This peculiar-looking stretcher, carried on a mule, was used by the military in rough terrain or if no ambulance was available (author's collection).

army didn't have vehicles expressly intended for transporting the sick and wounded. Wounded soldiers were transported in any manner that was feasible, including on a stretcher, on horseback, or in the back of a jolting wagon. One makeshift carrier was an Indian-type travois, which consisted of two poles lashed together, several feet apart, with a blanket between the two for the wounded man to lie on. One end of each pole was fastened to each side of a horse, while the other ends were dragged across the ground, creating what must have been a very bumpy ride.

In 1859 the secretary of war approved experimental models of two-wheeled and four-wheeled carriages that were intended specifically for transporting the sick and injured. The two-wheeled versions turned out to be unsuitable for transporting wounded men because they produced an unstable bouncing motion. Soldiers named them "gut-busters" because the ride they provided was harsh and jarring, and the vehicles frequently overturned, making injuries worse. The four-wheeled versions, equipped with folding bunks for transportation of the wounded, were commonly used in the West during the Indian Wars.

The two-wheeled units, however, turned out to be far more popular at army posts than the four-wheeled type. The two-wheelers were often commandeered by officers for personal and recreational transportation. The four-wheeled version was widely used in the West — if road conditions permitted.

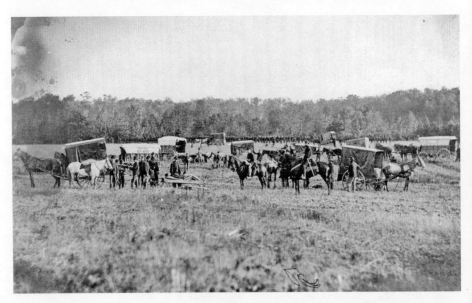

Both two-wheeled and four-wheeled ambulances, along with men on stretchers, are shown in this photograph of an infantry ambulance drill in 1864 (National Archives).

As well as being used for transportation of the wounded, they were also employed to transport army wives to and from remote army posts, and were available for the convenience of army generals.

The convoy that accompanied a large campaign into the field often included one or more ambulances. Being transported in one of these horse-drawn wagons, which had no springs to absorb the bumps, meant a long, jolting ride back to the nearest post for medical attention. The constant bouncing might aggravate severe wounds or broken bones enough to turn them into fatalities.

CHAPTER THREE

Filthy Towns and Filthy People

Several factors contributed to the spread of disease and illness in the Old West. Among them, haphazard sanitation, polluted water supplies, questionable personal hygiene, and a poor diet were often direct or contributing causes to many of the health challenges faced by frontier residents.

The smell of raw sewage, rotting garbage, decomposing animal carcasses, and unwashed bodies must have made an appalling combination in many of the early towns. The stench that hung over privies and unburied garbage had the impressive-sounding name of "mephitic effluvia." The nasty smell of decomposing corpses was thought to be a foul miasma, and burials usually took place with the least delay.

By the mid–1800s, large cities, such as Philadelphia and New York, had made substantial progress in sanitation and public health practices, but the state of public health in rural communities in the West continued to be essentially the same as it had been for the preceding hundred years in the East. The causes for diseases were mostly unknown, and the ancient theories of humors and miasmas were still popular ideas.[1] The name miasma was usually associated with swamps and the breeding grounds of malarial mosquitoes. As the presence of microbes and insect vectors had not yet been discovered, it seemed perfectly logical at the time that sickness arose as a result of exposure to some unknown, smelly part of the atmosphere.

Indeed, the foul smells that pervaded the atmosphere could easily be believed to be the origin of diseases. Physicians noted that many people fell ill during an epidemic without direct exposure to a sick person. Lacking proper knowledge, observers felt that the atmosphere was the common factor for transmission of diseases between victims of an epidemic. Objectionable smells, such as those arising from an outhouse or from rotted food, were intuitively felt to be corrupt and unpleasant, and, by association, dangerous.

Indirectly, this thinking paved the way for early sanitation. The reasoning followed the notion that if epidemics were transmitted by a miasma arising from filth and polluted water, then cleaning up the environment should remove the miasma and reduce the epidemics. The unrealized byproduct was that this clean-up also correctly removed rats, insects, bacteria, and other major carriers of disease, and eliminated the breeding grounds of mosquitoes and fleas. It was the right course of action, but for the wrong reasons.

Nevill Armstrong, one of the first to reach Dawson during the Klondike gold rush, reported that typhoid was rampant in the town. He later estimated that the number of those who died was about 120 a week — a figure that was probably high. Correct or not, his comment emphasized the rapid spread of disease that could occur in filthy towns.

As a contributing factor in disease epidemics, most of the population in the Old West lived in rural areas separated by long distances, rather than being concentrated in towns, as was more usual in the East. As a result, many of the children in the West were not exposed to common childhood diseases, such as measles, mumps, whooping cough, and smallpox. As these children grew into adulthood, people who were crowded together — for example, during a gold rush — were highly susceptible to catching all these diseases from each other. If one of these highly contagious diseases broke out in a mining camp, a crowded cattle town, an Indian village, or among the soldiers at a frontier fort, it could run rampant through the population. These childhood diseases were relatively uneventful among children and afterwards immunized them for life, but they could have a severe outcome if contracted by an adult. Measles, for example, was one of the childhood diseases that spread the most easily and could have fatal consequences in adults.

Sanitation in Town

A primary reason that disease was prevalent in the Old West was a lack of attention to general sanitation in many towns.

By 1850, hygienists in Britain had proven that the cleanup of water supplies, proper disposal of sewage, and the removal of garbage from the streets reduced many epidemics. American hygienists campaigned against filth and the sources of foul smells, but progress was slow. While sanitary practices did not attack the causes of diseases, sanitary disposal of sewage and cleaning up polluted water supplies reduced the occurrence of many illnesses by eliminating the sources in which they festered.

Sanitation in poorly-constructed mining and military camps, in particular, was crude. The problem had many aspects. For example, garbage disposal was sloppy. Before municipal dumps outside a town were established, pioneers often threw their garbage onto a pile in the back yard behind their houses, where it was left to rot. Piles of mule and horse manure, and other filth, accumulated in alleys. As a token improvement, trash was often taken by individuals to the edge of a town and dumped there. Later attempts to provide better sanitation resulted in a town dump that served the entire community, but it was often located within the town limits.

Mining and cattle towns attracted large concentrations of people without providing the appropriate sanitation. Streets were covered in litter — and worse. Spitting in public was common. Men commonly urinated wherever and whenever they needed to. The aroma of privies hung over the town in hot summer weather. Horse manure was everywhere on the streets, with clouds of flies buzzing over it in the summer. Stray dogs and wild animals trotted around, carrying rabies. Hog pens were typically built close to the owner's house, thus allowing the spread of filth and disease. Many times, hogs, chickens, cows, burros, and horses roamed the streets unrestrained, polluting wherever they went.[2] Some of this was deliberate. In an attempt to clean up early towns, pigs were occasionally turned loose on the streets to eat accumulated garbage.

Unpaved streets were filled with choking dust in summer and turned into a morass of mud in the winter. Streets were often littered with refuse, garbage, old food, and animal carcasses. One of the duties of the town marshal in the Old West was to dispose of dead animals lying in the street, as well as to act as a general street cleaner.

One darkly humorous example shows how bad the problem could become. During the 1890 gold rush to Dawson, in the Yukon Territory of Canada, a man named Arthur Walden wagered against local skeptics that he could cross the main thoroughfare without touching the muddy surface of the street. He won the bet by jumping from the carcass of one dead horse to another until he made it to the other side.

Mining camps were established in great haste as prospectors, miners, and merchants flooded to rich finds, all hoping to make easy money. The first gold seekers drawn out West from the East wanted to make their fortunes as quickly as possible and then return home. They were not interested in making a permanent place to live. As a result, if a gold strike played out, everyone abandoned a ramshackle infant town, moved on to the next promising strike, and started all over again.

Because buildings were hastily constructed, were located close together, and built of wood that was as dry as tinder, early towns were highly susceptible to fires. What might have been only minor fires often turned into major conflagrations because they were fueled by dynamite and kerosene that was stored in warehouses, shops, and other buildings. Most towns and mining camps had at least one fire in which the whole town was partially or completely burned down.

Cripple Creek, Colorado, suffered two devastating fires within days of each other in April 1896, which together burned most of the downtown area.

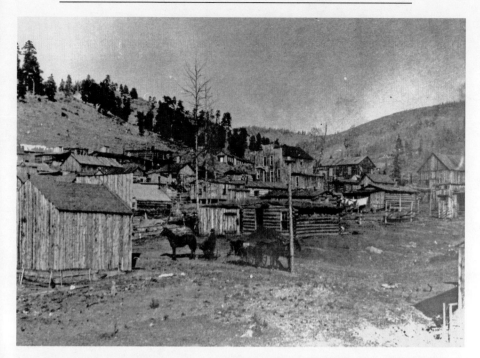

Early towns usually consisted of rough wooden shacks, such as in this unidentified mining town in Colorado, that were crowded hastily together, while the miners spent their time in the real business of looking for gold (Glenn Kinnaman, Colorado and Western History Collection).

What did not burn was inadvertently blown up by dynamite stored in a livery stable. Rebuilding started almost immediately and transformed the ramshackle burned-out buildings into a city of brick. A similar fire in 1899 in nearby Victor had the same results.

Over the Continental Divide to the southwest, a big fire in the town of Creede on June 5, 1892, burned out all the wooden shacks that lined the narrow streets, along with twelve bridges crossing the creek that ran through the center of town. Within a matter of hours the downtown area was reduced to a pile of smoldering ashes. Ten years later fire swept through the town again and wiped out two hotels and twenty houses.

Town fires were often deadly. On March 10, 1883, a fire near Brownsville, South Dakota, killed eleven men sleeping in the boarding house of the Hood and Scott lumber mill. Another four were seriously burned. To try to prevent such catastrophes, some towns employed a night watchman. His duty was not to police the town but to be on the lookout for fires in the night and raise the alarm in case of danger. Though fires were obviously a tragedy for the inhabitants of a town, they served a useful purpose by cleaning out accumulated garbage and filth, and removing rickety old buildings, thus paving the way for towns to be rebuilt in a more substantial manner.[3]

Town saloons, in particular, were notorious reservoirs of disease. Tobacco chewing was common, and men shot liquid streams of tobacco juice—complete with germs—whenever and wherever they felt the need. Cuspidors were placed along the front of the bar in saloons, but contemporary photographs show that the aim of most of the chewers was poor and the wooden floors were spattered with stains.

Sawdust was commonly spread on the floor in early saloons to soak up spilled drinks and poorly-aimed wads of tobacco intended for the spittoon. This practice, however, had other, more serious, consequences. When early mining towns were flooded with new inhabitants, there were not always enough hotel or boardinghouse rooms to accommodate all the new arrivals. To relieve the problem — or, more accurately, to profit from the shortage of beds— some saloons rented out their floors after they closed at night as sleeping space for those without rooms. The price for a night on the floor might

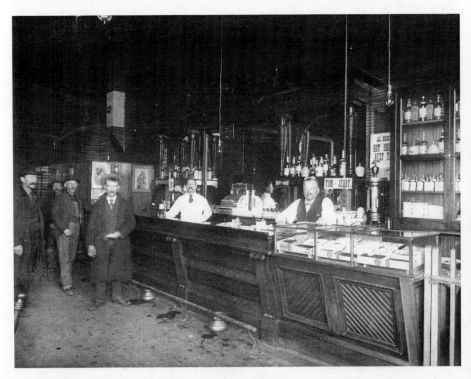

The accuracy of the aim of drinkers was not always good, as can be seen by the stains around the spittoons in this saloon. This practice led to the spread of lung diseases such as tuberculosis (Denver Public Library Western History Collection, X-660).

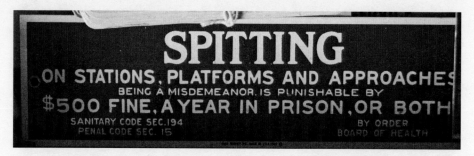

SPITTING
ON STATIONS, PLATFORMS AND APPROACHES
BEING A MISDEMEANOR, IS PUNISHABLE BY
$500 FINE, A YEAR IN PRISON, OR BOTH
SANITARY CODE SEC.194   BY ORDER
PENAL CODE SEC. 15   BOARD OF HEALTH

The common practice of spitting everywhere, such as on sidewalks, saloon floors, and railway platforms, was eventually outlawed to try to prevent the spread of diseases (author's collection).

be twenty-five cents. Due to the practice of poorly-aimed spitting, the sawdust on the floor became a reservoir for lung diseases such as tuberculosis or pneumonia, and was a serious hazard for those who slept on it.

Another health hazard of saloons was that whiskey found in hastily-improvised drinking establishments was often served out of tin cups or glasses that were not washed between customers, further contributing to the rapid and easy spread of disease.

The roadsides in and out of many towns were lined with animal carcasses. The terrain around early gold and silver mining towns was often so mountainous that the horses and mules used in teams as pack animals to carry gold and silver ore from the mines down to the smelters in the valleys died from exhaustion along the way. Trails that traversed steep mountain grades and high-altitude passes were so narrow that animals that were worked to death were unhitched from the rest of the team and pushed over the side of the trail. The carcasses lodged there, rotting and stinking in the hot summer sunshine. It was said — probably with some accuracy — that a blind man could find his way over many of the passes in the Colorado mining districts simply by following the smell of dead mules.

Sanitation at Home

The early log cabins and sod huts that were popular as dwellings in the Old West were not particularly sanitary places—either inside or out. In most instances they consisted of one large central room for living and sleeping. A stone fireplace at one end filled the room with smoke and greasy fumes from cooking, and coal oil lamps spewed out black smoke, all of which added to the overall aroma and created respiratory problems for the residents.

Beds were commonly stuffed with hay that was not changed as often as

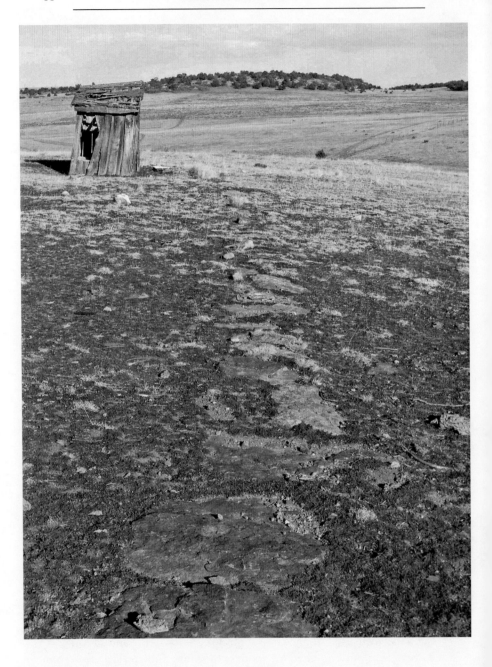

The pathway to the outdoor privy at night or in bad weather was not always appealing (author's collection).

it should have been. Mattresses were frequently the home of lice, which were derisively known as "seam squirrels." The soldier's mattress at early frontier army posts consisted of a cotton bag stuffed with straw, which was nicknamed "prairie feathers." The straw was supposed to be changed once a month.

Log homes and other early houses did not have screens on the windows or doors, thus allowing free access for insects. Flies, attracted to household smells, contributed to the spread of disease by landing on dining tables after crawling on animal and human waste. This method of transmission of disease was not understood until homeowners started using lime to sanitize their privies. Their first clue came when flies that entered through doors and windows left a white trail of lime as they crawled over the family food on the table.

The household toilet was a privy that consisted of a shallow hole in the ground in the back yard, with a small wooden building over it. Because houses were often built near a stream to provide a ready water supply, the house-

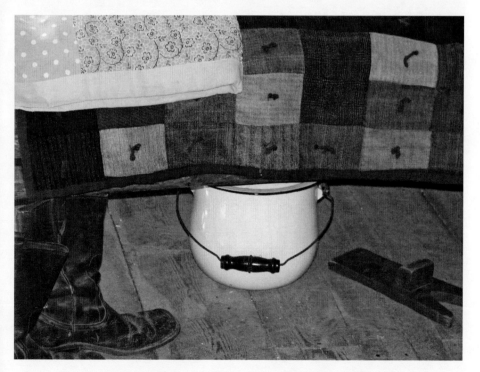

The answer was a chamber pot kept under the bed — perhaps emptied in the privy in the morning, perhaps simply thrown out onto the ground from an upstairs window (author's collection).

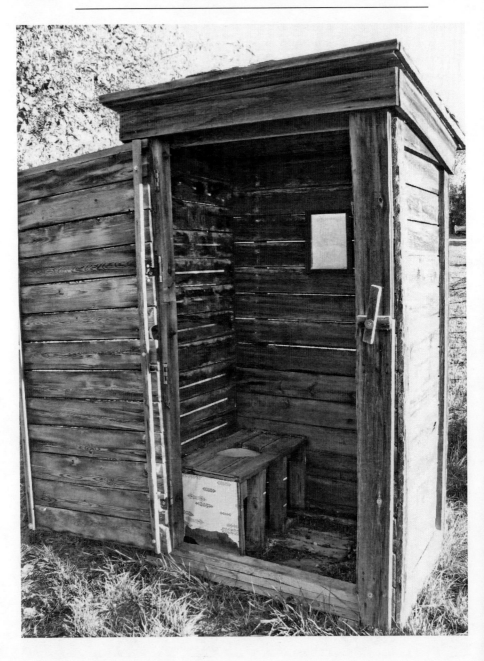

An outhouse was still an outhouse. Conventional pit-type of privy found behind the main house (author's collection).

hold privy often ended up too close to the stream, thus polluting the water supply for the owner and others downstream.

When the hole in the privy filled up, or the smell of excrement became too bad, the hole was covered over, a new one dug, and the outhouse moved over it again. In bad weather, or at night, householders used a chamber pot, also known colloquially as a "thundermug," inside the house, typically stored at the foot of the bed or underneath it. The contents of chamber pots were often simply thrown out of the window in the morning instead of being emptied into the privy.

Apart from disease, a further hazard of outhouses was the common presence of black widow spiders, which spun their webs in the dark areas underneath the wooden seat and were not afraid to bite the user on an exposed portion of their anatomy.

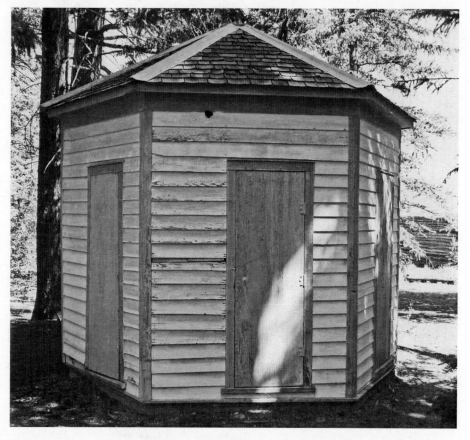

This curious six-sided outhouse offered no waiting for the guests at a six-room resort hotel in Colorado (author's collection).

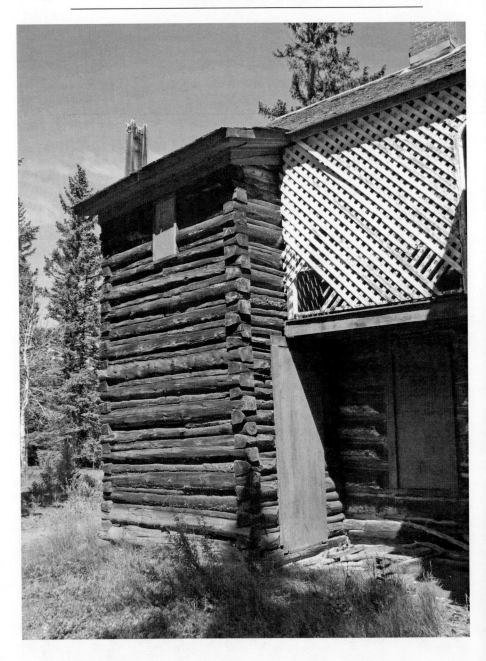

This unusual double-decker, stacked outhouse at the back of the Interlaken Hotel at Twin Lakes, Colorado, offered separate facilities for both floors of the hotel (author's collection).

Around the home, drinking cups, washbasins, and towels that were used by all of the family and any visitors contributed to the spread of disease. Drinking water was kept in a wooden bucket or barrel, and a communal cup, ladle, or tin dipper next to it was used by everyone. Families served food with the same spoons and forks that had just been in their mouths, thus propagating the spread of any disease present in any of them. Families washed their hands and faces in the same bowl, washed their dishes in the same water, and dried everything on the same towel. Hotels, schools, and other public establishments also used common drinking ladles and a common towel for everyone to wash their hands.

Cleaning dishes and eating utensils after a meal for soldiers in the field or cowboys on a cattle drive often consisted of merely wiping them off with leaves or sand, or perhaps rinsing them with the remains of the hot coffee that had accompanied the food. In many instances, plates and utensils were stored away without cleaning at all. As may be imagined, this unsanitary practice, plus questionable preparation of food out on the prairie or cattle trail, frequently led to diarrhea and dysentery.

Personal Hygiene

For many people raised on isolated ranches and farms without running water, and in early mining camps, ideas of personal hygiene were often less than adequate. Bathing was a difficult process and was not always a high priority. Consequently, many people did not wash themselves as frequently as they should have. Actually, daily bathing was not common at all among rural residents in the Old West during the second half of the nineteenth century. This unhygienic state was compounded by clothes

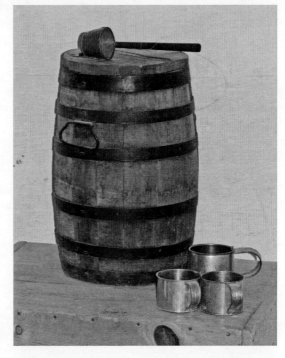

Disease was commonly spread by using a shared water dipper in a barrel of drinking water and drinking directly out of it, or by using unwashed tin cups that were stored nearby (author's collection).

that were often filthy from outside work, and might be caked with mud and cow manure.

Arthur Hertzler related one anecdote about a family he knew:

> All the boys were sewed into their clothes in the fall when cold weather approached. At bedtime, blankets were thrown on the floor and the young-sters lay down on them.... They woke in the morning all dressed.... In the spring the clothes were ripped off and the child saw himself, for the first time in a number of months.[4]

Bathing in log cabins and one-room houses was limited due to a lack of privacy and a lack of hot water. Primitive personal washing was accomplished instead with a cloth and cold or lukewarm water from a pitcher and wash-bowl. As late as the 1890s, small two-room miner's shacks in the mountains commonly had only one tin basin that was used both for washing dishes and bathing. Underneath the table was a "slop jar," which might be an old five-gallon oil can to receive the dirty water.

Women were generally more fastidious than men and tended to at least wash their faces. For women, Victorian reticence and crowded conditions in a small cabin meant that bathing might have to be accomplished while wear-ing a shift or nightgown, thus making the entire process a somewhat hap-hazard affair.

Until indoor bathrooms with running water became common, some peo-ple had never been wet all over from bathing or had taken a bath during their entire lives. Cowboys on the trail, and soldiers on Indian campaigns, tended more towards a brief splash on the face with water from a stream — or noth-ing at all. To further dampen any misplaced enthusiasm for a bath, regular bathing was thought to open up the pores of the skin and invite disease. When regular bathing became more common, the whole family washed in the same tub, using the same water. When bathrooms developed as a sepa-rate room in the house, they were rooms used only for bathing. Toilet facil-ities remained the outdoor privy.

Perfumes were not commonly used by women. Body odors were con-sidered normal and natural. Men might use some scented hair tonic when getting a haircut.

Personal hygiene among soldiers stationed in the West during the Indian Wars was often less than desirable. During the Civil War, it was said that an army on the march could be smelled before it was seen. The strong fragrance around encampments was sometimes called "the patriotic odor." Army reg-ulations required daily washing of hands and face, and feet twice a week. Men with a rural upbringing, who had to struggle to transport their water from a creek in a barrel, often didn't like to waste it on bathing and, as a con-sequence, didn't. Complete bathing was supposed to take place every week;

however, this did not always happen because of primitive conditions at some army posts. Water was usually at a premium at forts in the West and had to be transported from a well or nearby stream or river. After collecting enough water for drinking and cooking, most soldiers were not enthusiastic about collecting more just for bathing. A few forts had water piped to different buildings; however, easy access to good water did not occur at most forts until central water supplies were built in the 1890s.

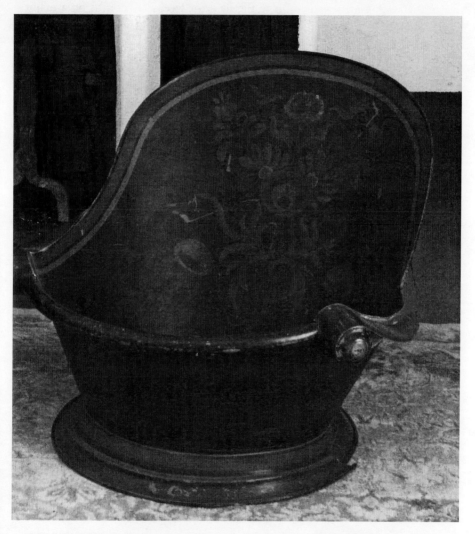

This elaborate bathtub, belonging to a well-to-do family, would be filled with water heated on the stove. The entire family would bathe in it, typically starting with father, then mother, then each child according to age (author's collection).

For cowboys and soldiers, jumping into a nearby creek or river during a warm summer evening to cool off — and bathe as a byproduct — was a popular practice. But in winter in the West, when rivers, ponds, and water barrels froze solid, the men omitted the practice. Because water was cold and facilities were lacking, the men often went for months without washing or bathing.

A similar lack of cleanliness applied to soldiers' clothes. Laundresses were available at military posts to wash the soldiers' uniforms every week, but when the men went off into the field for weeks or months on a major campaign, they might wear the same clothes for weeks at a time. If the clothes became too ripe, the men might wash them in a nearby creek during an overnight stop — probably in the same place where they also subsequently obtained their drinking water. Lacking suitable laundry utensils in the field, clothes were commonly washed in the same pots and kettles used for preparing food. Residues of soup, beans, and stew mixed with soap and whatever was washed out of the clothes, then went back into the next batch of food cooked in the pots, further spreading diarrhea and dysentery.

A lack of cleanliness of body and clothing meant that body lice (*Pedicu-*

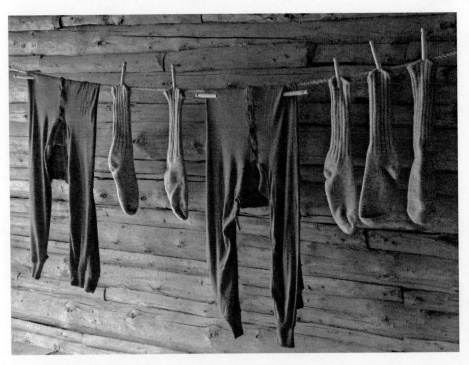

Soldiers were supposed to bathe and have their clothes, such as these socks and union suits, washed weekly. The primitive facilities for washing at many frontier forts meant that this didn't always happen (author's collection).

lus humanus corporis) were common. These small crawling insects, affectionately known as "graybacks" by soldiers, often carried typhus, which was a common affliction. After weeks in the field, soldiers found that the only way to completely get rid of lice might be to burn their clothing.

As well as the usual flies, lice, and assorted bedbugs, the cheaper lodgings in gold-rush San Francisco during the early 1850s were overrun with large gray rats. Many of the rodents were so large and voracious and bold that they attacked men while they were sleeping, biting off large pieces of flesh from ears and noses.

As the second half of the nineteenth century progressed and hygienists tried to introduce new practices of sanitation, they were joined by moral reformers who felt that personal cleanliness was an essential part of morality. Dirty clothing was considered to give off "impure vapors" that led to disease. As an extension of the humoral and miasma theories, the air trapped underneath bed covers was considered to be full of poisonous substances that had escaped through the pores of the skin during the night.

Contrary to the earlier opinion of Benjamin Rush, who felt that windows should be sealed tightly shut to prevent the entry of foul miasmas, moral reformers felt that bedroom windows should be wide open to fresh air. As late as 1874, one self-styled authority stated emphatically that "about 40 percent of all deaths are due to impure air."[5]

Pure Drinking Water

One of the most serious challenges for pioneers on the frontier was finding pure water to drink. One of the main causes for the spread of disease was contaminated drinking water because natural water supplies were frequently tainted with various diseases from previous users.

Richard Geoghegan joined the gold rush to the Klondike in 1897. When he was appointed court clerk in Fairbanks, Alaska, he wrote to his niece, "Water is a precious thing here, they have to go many miles to get it, because what they get in the river is evil and people cannot live on it; to tell the truth, it is mostly mud and dead dogs..."[6]

Pure water was not a sure thing anywhere in the Old West, and it was anyone's guess what pollutants might be found in the water. In 1880 the body of a murdered Mexican sheepherder was found in the water supply of Tombstone, Arizona. Unfortunately for those drinking the water, the body was there for several weeks before being found.

Obtaining an adequate supply of potable water was always a problem for settlers moving west. In the absence of a well, drinking water might have to come from a nearby creek or pond, and was stored in a barrel. Rain often

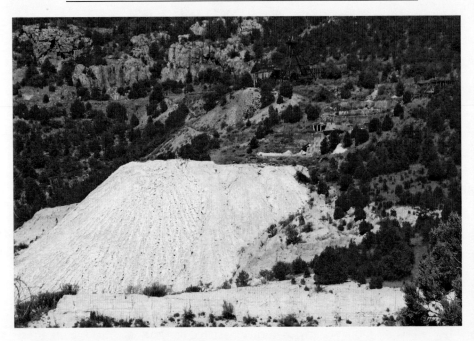

Huge dumps of waste material from ore processing mills, here near the mining town of Mogollon, New Mexico, left vast residues of toxic material that leached into the water table and created dust that was breathed into the lungs when the wind blew (author's collection).

fell in torrents on the Great Plains during the spring, but then ponds dried up quickly into mud lakes, and rain might not come again until the following spring. In the deserts of the Southwest, ponds might be stale and covered with scum. In the mountainous West, many ponds contained poisonous levels of chemicals that could be fatal when drunk. Men and animals often died after drinking water that was contaminated with toxic minerals, heavy metals, and alkali.[7]

During the early years of the mining rush to Virginia City and the Comstock in Nevada, the ground water was heavily polluted with soluble salts of arsenic, lead, and copper. As a result, water in the mines or streams that drained from the hillsides was highly poisonous. Miners that drank from innocent-looking streams suffered violent stomach cramps or, in the worst cases, died from drinking polluted water. One reputed preventative was to neutralize poisonous water by adding liberal amounts of whiskey—a solution (so to speak) that served many of the miners well.

There were few attempts at purifying water in the back country. Men simply dipped their canteens and coffee pots into lakes, rivers, streams, springs, ponds, and any other supplies of water that they found. When the men went to slake their thirst, often these were the same ponds that had been used by their oxen and horses a few minutes previously. Water polluted by animal or human feces led to diarrhea and serious intestinal infections, such as typhoid.

Army forts were generally constructed near rivers and streams in order to be close to water supplies. Though builders eventually learned to avoid swampy areas because of the danger of mosquitoes and the diseases they carried, there were no methods of purifying drinking water. Likewise, settlers who camped near convenient rivers and springs suffered from diseases left by previous wagon trains. Soldiers noted that coffee tasted "different" when cavalry horses were watered upstream from where they drew out their drinking water. It was not until the late 1880s that the larger army posts redesigned and rebuilt their water supplies, along with their system of sewage disposal, using sanitary guidelines.

In the East, reforms had led to the creation of sanitary municipal water supplies. Philadelphia built a water supply in 1830, New York followed in 1842, and Boston in 1843. Towns in the West were slower to follow. Crested Butte, Colorado, for example, didn't complete their system until 1883. Leadville, Colorado, didn't install its municipal water system until 1879, even though the population by then had grown to more than 20,000 inhabitants. Perversely, the city didn't install a municipal sewer system to remove their waste water until 1886. Even then the system only served businesses and a few homes in the center of the city.

In the West, before the development of sanitary water supplies, municipal water usually came from a communal well or nearby stream. However, privies and stables were often inappropriately located where they would drain into the water supply. In Denver, refuse and sewage from hotels, restaurants, and saloons, along with the waste from laundries, slaughter yards, homes, stables, and privies, went directly into the South Platte River, which ran through the center of town. Water was drawn out of the river for drinking, washing, and other household uses.

Western towns usually grew too fast for local authorities to provide adequate water supplies and sewage disposal. As settlements became more established and towns grew, most water holes, springs, streams, and shallow wells became polluted. In growing towns or out on the ranch, wells used for drinking water were typically located near a stable, the privy, or the kitchen drain. Garbage left outside to rot often ended up near wells. Wastewater from bathing and washing dishes was thrown outside the front door, often in the general direction of the well, where it percolated down into the ground and back into the drinking water supply. In some towns, wastewater from houses was piped directly into the streets and left to drain away haphazardly. Even under the best conditions, drainage was carried away in open ditches.

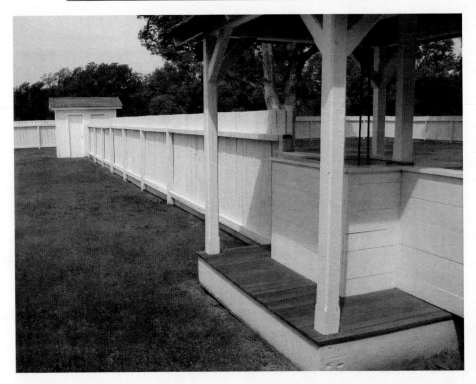

The household well for drinking water (right foreground) was often located too close to the privy (left background), resulting in underground leakage of the privy contents into the well, starting a cycle of disease (author's collection).

Under these circumstances, settlers in the Old West often created their own sources of water contamination when disease agents leaked into the wells. Goldfield, Nevada, suffered a severe typhoid epidemic in the early 1900s. The cause was found to be contamination of private water wells by untreated sewage. An outbreak of typhoid in 1904 in the mining town of Leadville, Colorado, was traced to sewage deposited in an unlined settling tank that was several feet above the pipes that supplied the city's drinking water. One of the pipes was cracked and, as a result, raw sewage seeped into the drinking water distribution system.

Some towns discharged untreated sewage directly into nearby rivers and streams. This water was then used for drinking water by other towns downstream, with little attempts at purification. In 1904, for example, the Colorado State Board of Health reported that an outbreak of typhoid at the Camp Bird ore mill above Ouray, Colorado, was followed very rapidly by a similar outbreak in the town of Montrose, which was located forty miles or so downstream.

Diet

A poorly-balanced diet, consisting primarily of beans and salt pork, bacon, and ham, for soldiers, cowboys, and prospectors in mining camps, and a tendency to fry all food, resulted in frequent stomach distress and illness.[8] A diet high in meat, such as deer, elk and beef, combined with a lack of fresh vegetables and fruit, tended to plug the old miners up. Old bottles from laxative preparations, such as Duffee's Fifty-Fifty Laxative Tonic Tablets and Upjohn's Phenolax Wafers, are commonly found in trash heaps in old mining and ghost towns, indicating the extent of the problem.

One folk remedy for an upset stomach was to drink tea made from mint leaves or to chew directly on the leaves themselves. Mint was thought to aid the digestion, and hence led to the common modern practice and popularity of eating an after-dinner mint.

A working man's diet leaned heavily towards fats and starch (such as potatoes, bread, and beans) in order to provide the energy to do heavy work all day. These provided plenty of calories, but not a balanced diet. As one example of the lack of understanding of diet, at one time New York City banned the sale of tomatoes because they were thought to be poisonous.

Food was often contaminated. As a result, typhoid, dysentery, and diarrhea due to diet were common and often fatal. Adding to the dietary imbalance, the frequent use of alcohol — wine, whiskey, and beer — led to upset stomachs and other digestive problems. Drinking was popular with meals. Alcohol was commonly drunk with meals, after meals, and between meals.

Army rations frequently contributed to the semi-permanent diarrhea and dysentery endured by many soldiers. Hardtack, a rock-hard flour-and-water biscuit about three inches square, was often green and moldy. Improper storage allowed hardtack to become infested with maggots and weevils, a brown insect about an eighth of an inch long that could bore into the hardest biscuit.

Soldiers learned to dip hardtack into hot coffee to drown the bugs, then skimmed them off the surface of the brew. Another technique to defeat the bugs was to fry hardtack in bacon grease to kill weevils and maggots. When fried to the point of charring, hardtack was thought to be good for strengthening weak bowels. Army bread did not have the digestive problems associated with hardtack because it was baked fresh daily, though the flour barrels were often infested with weevils, worms, mouse droppings, and maggots.

Too much meat also led to gastric upsets. The staple of the soldier's diet was salt pork, also called "sowbelly," which was pork packed in barrels, with salt as a preservative. The pork was frequently green, rancid, and slimy after long storage. Before cooking, the meat had to be soaked for a lengthy period of time to remove the salt. If this was not done correctly, further stomach troubles resulted. Troops in the field might tie a chunk of meat to a rope and put it in a running stream overnight to try to reduce the brine content and make the meat more palatable. Salt beef, also known derisively to the soldiers as "salt horse," was prepared in a similar fashion.

CHAPTER FOUR

Common Diseases

The lack of proper sanitation in the Old West resulted in widespread disease. Cholera, typhoid, smallpox, malaria, typhus, and yellow fever struck with frightening regularity. The microorganisms responsible for these diseases required high population densities so that they could thrive in a reservoir of susceptible individuals. Diarrhea and dysentery occurred frequently among emigrants in wagon trains headed West, and scurvy was common after months of a diet of salt pork and flapjacks. Estimates are that as many as one-third of the men who journeyed West suffered from various diseases. Many of these diseases struck without warning and overcame their victims with surprising speed. The result of disease, when combined with the poor diet that left many pioneers in a weakened condition, could be deadly.

Historically, many of the diseases of mankind originated with animals. Tuberculosis and smallpox originally came from cattle; influenza from pigs and ducks. The common cold jumped to man from horses. Measles originally came from a mutated form of canine distemper that had its source in dogs and cattle.

The nineteenth-century term used for disease that arose from indirect contact, such as measles and scarlet fever, was "contagion." The term "infection" was used for those diseases that required direct physical contact, such as smallpox and syphilis.

Sick individuals (for example, those with typhus and measles) were thought to produce poisonous miasmas. These invisible poisons that floated through the air were also called "ferments" because they were assumed to follow the same fermenting process of degeneration as spoiled milk and rotten fruit. The concept of insects, such as mosquitoes and fleas, being agents of disease transmission was ridiculed.

One army report showed that out of 1,800 cases treated at sick call, 1,550 were for disease and 250 were for wounds, accidents and other injuries. Out of the cases treated, thirteen men died — eight from disease and five from other causes.

Cholera

One of the most notorious killers on the frontier was cholera, a severe gastrointestinal infection transmitted primarily through contaminated water supplies. Major cholera epidemics raged through the United States in 1832, 1849, and 1866. Cholera typically spread rapidly among people living together in relatively large concentrations, such as in an emigrant wagon train headed for California, a railroad construction camp, a frontier town, an Indian tribe, or a frontier fort full of soldiers. The true cause, a bacterium that was spread to water and food from the feces of an infected person, was not understood at the time.

The 1849 outbreak in the United States that struck travelers on the Oregon Trail was the end of a massive epidemic of Asiatic cholera that had spread around the world, starting in 1846. The disease traveled from India, across China, to Russia, and then marched inexorably eastwards. In 1848 it passed through most of the countries of Europe, including Germany, France, and England, taking a million lives in the process. In areas where severe outbreaks occurred, at least half of those who contracted the disease died.

Before modern sanitation and water purification practices became widespread, cholera was a serious problem. In the mid–1800s, even the cause of the disease was unknown. Settlers on a wagon train whose members contracted the disease could only provide a few supportive measures and hope for the best.

Some authorities stated categorically that cholera attacked only those who were intemperate and had a dissolute way of life. Doctors in the East noted that cholera seemed to strike in areas of cities where filth and squalor prevailed, but that reinforced the general view that the disease was associated with degenerate people and their drunken lifestyles. It was with some surprise, therefore, that in the mid–1850s doctors noted that even respectable ladies in nice neighborhoods were falling victim to the disease. Many doctors believed that cholera was not contagious, but they had a hard time persuading others to nurse the sick or bury the dead.

The incubation period for cholera lasted anywhere from a few hours to four or five days, but the disease could be frightening in its speedy onset. Some who caught the disease went into shock and died within two or three hours. Early symptoms were uncontrollable watery diarrhea, fever, and vomiting.

Contracting the illness resulted in painful muscular cramps and an unquenchable thirst, then overwhelming diarrhea and violent vomiting that completely dehydrated the victim. Collapse followed in a short time. The final stage lasted from a few hours to a few days before the victim died. In the disease's worst incarnation, an individual could be apparently healthy in the morning, collapse without warning at noon, and die in convulsions by nightfall.

As the disease progressed, the victim could lose so much fluid that their body weight dropped by as much as one-fourth. The end was reached when the disturbance of water and electrolytes in the body went so far out of balance that the victim's heart gave out. The classic symptoms of dehydration as the end approached were puckered blue lips and a hideous shriveled face. Today cholera is treated with antibiotics, and replacement of the body's fluids and electrolytes that have been depleted by the constant diarrhea.

Westerners first encountered cholera in 1817 on the Ganges Delta of India when an outbreak killed 9,000 British troops.[1] Infected individuals, who traveled and traded around the world, soon spread the disease to the United States, and cholera ran rampant in New Orleans, Chicago, and Detroit. Between 1832 and 1834, more than 200,000 Americans died from cholera. New Orleans was particularly prone to disease because the town was built on swampy ground, it had no public water supply, its sources of drinking water were below sea level, and most of the city had poor drainage. Attempts to control the spread of cholera consisted of burning sulfur, pine tar, or gunpowder. Other preventatives were spreading lime and washing the inside walls of buildings with vinegar.

Cholera outbreaks came and went with no apparent cause, and there was no clear idea of how it spread. Some thought that it was carried by miasmas—the traditional culprit of gaseous exhalations or terrible smells. Their view was that anyone who breathed these gases was in danger. Due to this type of misguided thinking, researchers did not pursue the real culprit. Because the disease and its symptoms were related to the intestinal tract, they should have realized that the real cause was something that was swallowed rather than something that was inhaled.

Some believed that cholera was related to either a lack or excess of electricity in the air. Others linked it to an excess of nitrogen or a deficiency of oxygen. One fanciful conjecture posited that cholera was caused by a lack of ozone in the atmosphere. The supposed cure was to take sulfur pills, a fad which became very popular for a while.

With great originality, doctors in Alabama and Philadelphia thought that purging was the answer and, during their great epidemics, treated cholera with frequent enemas. Another cure was a medicine made from cinnamon bark, cloves, and gum guaic dissolved in brandy. A third was a mixture of laudanum, spirits of camphor, and rhubarb. All of these "cures" had a decided purgative effect and created further dangerous fluid loss in an already dehydrated patient. Other attempted cures ranged from drinking laudanum to covering food with hot pepper sauce. Dr. Burchard treated cholera victims on the Santa Fe Trail in 1849 with enemas made from a combination of sugar of lead (lead acetate), laudanum, and gum arabica — but to no avail. Some wagon trains lost two-thirds of their people.

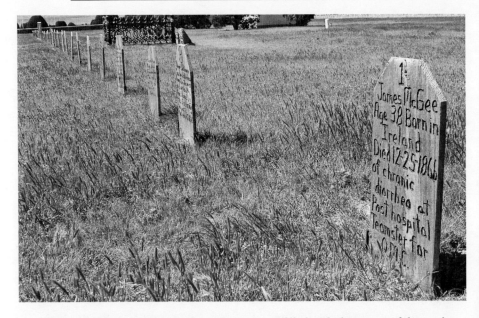

The post cemetery at Fort Wallace, Kansas, was filled with the graves of those who died from disease. On the right is a dysentery victim, 1866 (author's collection).

During the mass migrations of 1849 and 1850 along the Oregon Trail from either St. Joseph or Independence, Missouri (the main jumping-off points), to Sutter's Fort in California, cholera killed countless thousands. When wagons started rolling west in 1849 the cause of cholera was unknown. Wagon trains often camped unknowingly at creeks that were fouled with cholera. Emigrants on the Oregon Trail were warned to purify their drinking water during the trip, but most did not bother.

So little was known about cholera and its spread that one theory proclaimed that dried beans were responsible for the disease. As a safety precaution, many emigrant wagon trains discarded all their stocks of beans alongside the trail. Of course, the real problem was unseen microorganisms that lurked in water.

The 1849 migration across the Great Plains to California and Oregon also carried cholera to the Indians. The disease raged across the plains well into the 1850s. The Cheyenne called cholera the "Big Cramps" when it wiped out about half of their tribe. The spread of disease also resulted from the Indians' own doing. Indians often raided the graves of migrants who had died of cholera along the trail in order to recover clothes from the bodies. As they did so, they often unknowingly infected themselves with the disease.

The first stretch of the Oregon Trail, from Independence to Ft. Laramie, Wyoming, was littered with graves. This was a journey of 635 miles, which

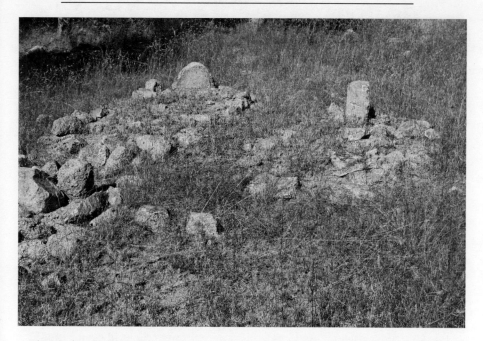

Those who died along the emigrant trails from St. Louis or Independence to the West were often buried in rough graves covered only with a pile of rocks to keep away wild animals (author's collection).

took between thirty and forty days. Francis Parkman, who traveled west from St. Joseph on the Oregon Trail with several companions in 1846, noted, "Sometimes we passed the grave of one who had sickened and died on the way." He added ominously, "The earth was usually torn up, and covered thickly with wolf-tracks ... [but] some had escaped this violation."[2] When a soldier from the Missouri volunteers died along the Santa Fe Trail in 1847, his comrades covered his grave with rocks and planted prickly pear cactus on top of it to try and prevent the wolves from digging up his body.

A major supply and restocking point for travelers along the Oregon Trail was Fort Laramie in present-day Wyoming. As a result, a further disease hazard specifically around this fort was a huge garbage dump that accumulated behind the main buildings, as travelers abandoned equipment and supplies that they didn't need. Large piles of discarded food rotted in the hot sun and attracted flies, rodents, and other carriers of disease.

If travelers made it beyond Ft. Laramie, the incidence of cholera was reported to be lower. Reasons given at the time were that the altitude was higher and the water fresher. In reality, the decrease was probably because there were fewer wagon trains on the last parts of the trails beyond Fort Bridger, where the Oregon Trail headed north through the Oregon Territory, and the California Trail continued west to Sacramento. Fewer wagons resulted in less congestion around water holes and less contamination of streams. Cholera was still a possibility on the final leg of the California Trail, but the threat was definitely decreased.

Even though the threat of cholera was reduced on the western parts of the trails, other dangers were present. In the Black Hills of South Dakota, for example, many of the water holes were tainted with alkali. Oxen — and unwary travelers — who drank the poisonous water often died, adding a border of rotting, disease-infested corpses to the following few miles of the trail.

When the emigrants finally reached the promised land of California, they found some relief from cholera, and, for the first couple of years, the gold camps seemed to be free of the disease. But then cholera struck San Francisco in October 1850, following the arrival of the ship *Carolina*, which had experienced a severe cholera outbreak on the trip north from Panama. Fourteen of the twenty-two passengers who contracted the disease died. The epidemic of cholera then swept up into the Sierra Nevada Mountains and through the gold camps. The major cities in California, San Francisco and Sacramento, suffered the most from the outbreak, but even the smaller gold camps, such as Coloma, Jamestown, Marysville, and Placerville, experienced deaths from cholera. Lesser epidemics swept through the gold camps in 1852 and 1854.

It was not until 1883 that German bacteriologist Robert Koch identified the real cause of cholera as the bacillus *Vibrio comma* (also known as *Vibrio cholerae*), which attacked the intestine and was then excreted in human feces.

Diarrhea and Dysentery

In the mid–1800s, diarrhea and dysentery were often confused with each other and thought to be the same problem. With a poor understanding of the causes of disease, doctors were not able to distinguish between the two. Indeed, the name "cholera" was sometimes given to any dysentery or diarrhea, even if that specific disease was not the cause.

Medically speaking, diarrhea is frequent and uncontrolled evacuations of the bowel that is symptomatic of some form of intestinal disorder. Dysentery, on the other hand, is the name applied to a collection of intestinal diseases that are characterized by inflammation of the bowel wall and are caused by various viral or bacterial infections, or parasites in the intestines. Though diarrhea and dysentery arose from various causes, the commonest were improper preparation of food, and poor or absent sanitation practices.

Dysentery in the Old West often resulted from toxic organisms, such as the ameba *Entamoeba histolytica*, swallowed in tainted water or food, such as spoiled meat. Salmonella, giardia, and staphylococci were other contributors. The result was violent diarrhea, accompanied by severe abdominal cramps and frequent stools of blood, pus, and mucus due to internal bleeding and breakdown of the intestinal wall. Because of these symptoms, dysentery was known colloquially on the frontier as the "flux" or "bloody flux." One surgeon reported that a mixture of mercury, chalk, Dover's powder, and quinine administered several times a day seemed to be successful.

As Francis Parkman delicately put it in 1846, "I had been slightly ill for several weeks, but on the third night after reaching Fort Laramie a violent pain awoke me and I found myself attacked by the same disorder that occasioned such heavy losses to the army on the Rio Grande. In a day and a half I was reduced to extreme weakness, so that I could not walk without pain or effort." Not having any real options, his cure was simple; he did nothing. "Having no medical adviser, nor any choice of diet, I resolved to throw myself upon Providence for recovery, using, without regard for the disorder, any portion of strength that might remain to me." In spite of weakness and pain, Parkman carried on with his daily business as best he could. But at some cost. He added, "I could scarcely keep my seat on horseback."[3]

By the end of the summer he was not much better. "For two days past I had been severely attacked by the same disorder which had so greatly reduced my strength when at the mountains; at this time I was suffering not a little from pain and weakness." Upon consulting a doctor, Parkman went through the following exchange: "'Your system, sir, is in a disordered state,' said he, solemnly, after a short examination. I inquired what might be the particular species of disorder. 'Evidently a morbid action of the liver,' replied the medical man; 'I will give you a prescription.'" The doctor gave him some medicine. "'What is it?' said I. 'Calomel,' said the doctor."[4]

This desire to purge and otherwise mistreat the bowels resulted in another cure that consisted of an enema made from a mixture of milk, slippery elm, oil, molasses, salt, and laudanum. A better treatment was opium or paregoric by mouth, both of which slowed down intestinal motility and reduced output.

In the military, during the Indian Wars in the West of the second half of the nineteenth century, when disease, living conditions, and nutrition often caused diarrhea, few attempts were made to distinguish between diarrhea and dysentery. The condition could become chronic. James Marshall, a soldier at Camp Verde, Arizona, contracted malaria in the summer of 1870. His diarrhea lasted for over two years until he was discharged in March of 1873, having never fully recovered. In 1893 the Army Medical Corps reported that almost 10 percent of frontier troops were suffering from diarrhea and dysentery.

It was not until the techniques of bacteriology were sufficiently advanced in the late 1870s and 1880s that progress could be made in determining the true culprits of these diseases. The cause of bacillary dysentery, for example, was not explained until 1898, when Kiyoshi Shiga discovered the *Shigella* bacterium.

Diphtheria

Diphtheria was one of the most terrible childhood diseases of the Old West and was estimated to be responsible for 25 percent of all childhood deaths. Arthur Hertzler noted in his biography that eight out of nine children in one family of his playmates died from diphtheria during one ten-day period.[5]

Major outbreaks of diphtheria occurred in the United States in 1863, 1874, 1882, and 1889. The disease could ravish an entire community, such as occurred during a severe outbreak in Park City, Utah, in 1880. It was not uncommon for half-a-dozen people a week to die when a small town was infected.

Transmission of diphtheria resulted from breathing air contaminated by the coughs or sneezes of an infected person, or through the unsanitary practice of spitting on the sidewalk or floor that was prevalent in the Old West. Transmission was also through direct contact with an infected carrier or from articles contaminated by a diphtheria patient. Eventually the disease developed a tough, whitish-gray slime in the throat that could suffocate the patient. After about a week, death commonly resulted from toxins released by the bacteria that caused the disease.

Because of the lack of understanding of the causes of disease and a lack of ability to differentiate between many of them, diphtheria and scarlet fever were considered by many to be the same disease. The symptoms were similar, and the methods of transmission were the same, though scarlet fever often involved death due to damage of the kidneys and brain.

Diphtheria was also known as "throat distemper," "putrid throat distemper," "bladder in the throat," and by the impressive-sounding name of "epidemical eruptive military fever." Victims developed a fever and suffered from a throat that became swollen and flecked with white. Another symptom was profound weakness. Treatment was to swab the throat with silver nitrate solution or tincture of iodine. Victims of the disease gargled with potassium chlorate or hydrogen peroxide.

Corynebacterium diphtheriae, the bacterium that caused the disease, was identified in 1884 by Edwin Klebs and Friedrich Löffler, but it was not until 1890 that effective diphtheria antitoxins were developed by Emil Behring. Antitoxin treatment rapidly pushed the mortality rate down from 40 percent to about 5 percent. Immunization drastically reduced the incidence of the disease by the early 1900s.

Malaria

Malaria, which was brought by early settlers to America, was the most common and deadly of all the frontier diseases. Malaria was particularly prevalent around the Mississippi Valley. The disease was common in Indiana, Illinois, Ohio, Wisconsin, and Missouri. The high country of the Southwest and the Rockies was relatively free from malaria, but it was rampant in the valleys and lowlands where settlers claimed land along streams and rivers. Many of the settlers carried the malaria parasite with them and infected local mosquitoes, who spread the disease further as they bit into new victims.

The causes were not understood, as the following extract from a medical manual that was contemporary with the Santa Fe Trail illustrates: "This disease is also caused by debility, produced by a poor, watery diet, damp houses, evening dews, lying upon damp ground, watchings, fatigue, depressing passions of the mind, &c."[6]

Because malaria was thought to originate with the foul air of a miasma, the name came from combining the Italian words "mal" and "aria," meaning "bad air." The disease was also known as "ague," "bilious fever," "autumnal fever," or "miasmal fever." Symptoms of the disease were alternating chills, fever, and sweats, along with aches, pains, and other uncomfortable symptoms. The names "fever" and "ague" were frequently applied indiscriminately to categorize any chills or fever, though often the real cause was malaria. The shaking produced by the chills that racked the sufferer gave malaria the simple name of "the shakes."

Malaria was caused by parasites that were transmitted to humans through the bite of an infected female mosquito.[7] Following a bite, the malarial parasites entered the bloodstream, where they matured and propagated within red blood cells. Symptoms developed when the parasites multiplied to the point that they ruptured the cell wall and flowed into the bloodstream again. Due to periodic eruption of successive generations of parasites, malarial fever had a recurrent nature and incapacitated the victim at various intervals. Because of this, malaria received the alternate names of "intermittent fever" and "recurrent fever."[8]

The treatment for malaria was to take quinine, a clear, bitter liquid derived from bark of the *Cinchona officinalis* tree, which grew in many tropical countries, typically South America. Quinine did not cure malaria, but it did control it. Because of its South American origins, quinine was also known as "Peruvian Bark." It was occasionally called "Jesuit Bark" or "Jesuit Powder" because Jesuit priests played a major role in introducing chinchona to Europe.

Because chinchona bark was collected in the jungles of South America, it was hard to obtain and expensive. Peruvian bark was also, unfortunately, difficult to administer as a medicine. It was bulky, it often produced nausea, and it had a purgative action that tended to produce diarrhea. In addition, calculating the dosage required was difficult, because the amount given depended on the strength and quality of the quinine in that particular bark. By the time the emigrants crossed the West, these problems were partially solved because a pure form of quinine had been isolated by pharmacists Pierre Joseph Pelletier and Joseph Bienaimé Caventou in Paris in 1820. The use of quinine was slow to be adopted in the United States because many doctors preferred to stick to the so-called "heroic" measures.

Though a course of treatment for malaria became available with quinine, the true cause of the disease, a parasite, was not discovered until 1880 by French physician Charles Louise Alphonse Laveran. Even after that, the method of transmission of the disease remained a mystery until 1897, when Ronald Ross discovered that the malaria parasite *Plasmodium* was transmitted by the *Anopheles* mosquito.

The experience of travelers on the Santa Fe Trail was common to all the emigrants to the West. Crossing Kansas along the Arkansas River, they encountered many mosquitoes when wagon trains camped in low places beside rivers, streams, and ponds in order to conveniently obtain drinking water. As more wagon trains traveled to the West, malarial mosquitoes infected the travelers, who in turn infected more mosquitoes, who then infected new travelers, until the problem became endemic to an area.

This was not a new problem, and the Arkansas River had always been a major source of malaria. At one point in 1827, when Fort Leavenworth, Kansas, was under construction, seventy-seven soldiers became ill with malaria at the same time. In 1858, the post surgeon at Fort Kearny, Nebraska, said that he had never seen so much malaria and so many fevers as were occurring among emigrant wagon trains passing the fort. Camp Verde, Arizona (originally named Camp Lincoln), was built as a military outpost in 1865 near the Verde River. Over the next few years the occurrence of malaria among the soldiers was so bad that in 1870 the army decided to move the camp a mile further away from the river. In 1897 the Army Medical Corps reported that malaria was causing illness in a little over 9 percent of frontier troops.

Malaria was a constant problem on the way to the California gold fields in 1849 and the early 1850s. A particularly virulent strain of malaria that struck those who traveled across the Isthmus of Panama was "Chagres fever." A medical survey of the area indicated that the life expectancy of the local natives was only about twenty years, with malaria being one of the prime causes of

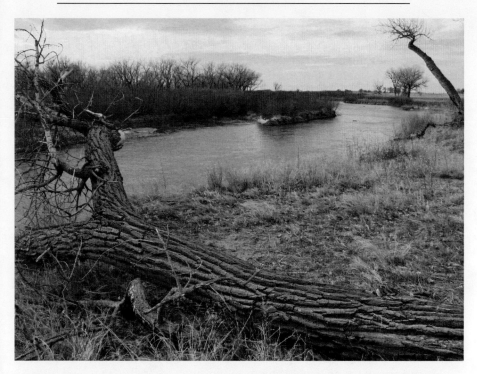

The Arkansas River, shown here in eastern Colorado alongside the Santa Fe Trail, was a breeding ground for mosquitoes that spread malaria among travelers who camped close to water supplies at night (author's collection).

death. The surgeon for the Panama Railroad, Dr. Chauncey Griswold, in line with medical thinking of the time, believed that the fever was due to foul miasmas from the surrounding swamps and recommended that travelers sleep with their doors and windows tightly closed, in spite of the oppressive heat. He also recommended doses of fifteen grains of quinine, an amount so large that it probably loosened the teeth and contributed to kidney damage.

The journey to California across the Isthmus of Panama took about five weeks; thus, malaria picked up along the Chagres River might not strike until after the traveler had reached California. After the Forty-Niners arrived in California, malaria was a constant source of death in the Central Valley towns into the late nineteenth century.

Scurvy

One of the persistent and frequent killers in the American West was scurvy. It was caused by a lack of vitamin C, even though the disease was easily treated by adding fresh fruits and vegetables to the diet. Scurvy occurred commonly in the West when no fresh vegetables or fruits were available, particularly during the winter months.

As early as 1754, British physician James Lind wrote that experience had shown that scurvy, and its horrible symptoms, could be prevented by adding vegetables or ripe fruit, such as oranges or lemons, to the diet. Though this was well-known at the time, it was also soon forgotten, and the cure for scurvy was "rediscovered" and "lost" several times.

Symptoms of scurvy included loosening of the teeth due to a loss of calcium in the jawbone, bleeding gums, wounds that wouldn't heal, and a loss of muscle tissue. If untreated, scurvy could lead to death due to degeneration of the heart muscles and subsequent massive internal bleeding. Cowboys and cavalry soldiers, in particular, who had scurvy and who spent long hours in the saddle, tended to develop bleeding sores on their backsides and thighs where pressure from the leather seats caused skin hemorrhages.

Those bound for Oregon and California in emigrant wagon trains suffered from scurvy because they primarily ate salt meat, corn, and dried beans, and no fresh vegetables. Pioneers were warned to take precautions, but scurvy still ranked as one of the most serious causes of sickness and death in the West. Knowledgeable travelers carried preserved fruit or citric acid with them, or made salads using green plants that they found growing wild along the way. In spring and summer, wild onions found along the trail were a good source of vitamin C.[9] So were the plants bistort and lamb's quarter. Mountain sorrel was high in vitamin C and was used by Native Americans to prevent scurvy.

Outbreaks of scurvy were frequent among gold prospectors and miners in the California gold fields due to their diet of greasy meat and beans. Because of this poor nutrition, the health of many of the men was broken by curable diseases, such as malaria and scurvy. In this weakened state, cholera, dysentery, and various respiratory problems could kill a miner, and, indeed, many died from these diseases.

Dr. Stillman of Sacramento described one unusual remedy for scurvy. This cure consisted of burying victims up to their necks in the earth, thereby hoping to soak up the healing powers of the soil. In the case of a large outbreak, one or two men were left in the open to assist those who were buried and protect them from marauding wild animals.

Soldiers at army posts on the Western frontier commonly had scurvy in winter, when fresh vegetables were not available. Because of primitive conditions at Fort Phil Kearny in Wyoming, scurvy was rampant in the winter of 1867. As a result, many of the men became weak and lost their teeth. The post surgeon finally cured the disease by sending the men out to find wild onions when they bloomed in the spring.

A soldier's meat ration was augmented by the appropriate amounts of beans, peas, or vinegar to try to combat scurvy; but, nonetheless, post hospital wards were often full of sick men, and some died of the disease. Because fresh vegetables were not provided as a part of issued rations, each company maintained a small garden on post during the summer to provide fresh vegetables. Depending on the tastes of the men, gardens could supply lettuce, cucumbers, potatoes, radishes, and squash. In winter, one alternative was to use desiccated vegetables, which came in the form of a dried, compressed mix of different vegetables that resembled a small brick in size and texture. A chunk of this brick was simmered in boiling water to form an unappetizing type of thick soup.

Smallpox

Smallpox, caused by the *Variola major* virus, was the real plague of the Old West. Smallpox was one of most contagious diseases known to man, was one of the worst and most dreaded, and was often fatal. The disease was caused by a virus transmitted by direct contact with an infected person or some item of their clothing. The disease could also be spread if the virus was coughed or sneezed into the air and inhaled by others.

The disease was so contagious that people did not want to go near bodies of smallpox victims for fear of catching the disease themselves. When cowboy Johnnie Blair died of smallpox in Tombstone, Arizona, in 1882, no one would carry him to his grave to bury his body. Finally, another cowboy threw a rope over his feet and dragged him to the gravesite.

Smallpox was an old disease of mankind and had existed since before the Roman Empire. It probably made its first appearance around 10,000 B.C. The symptoms were similar to influenza. The disease caused chills, abdominal pain, vomiting, and high fever, then a red rash appeared across the body, followed by crusty skin eruptions that caused severe itching all over the body. These pus-filled blisters swelled and then turned into scabs. Scratching to try to alleviate the itching led to secondary infections that were frequently fatal. If the patient lasted through this stage, the scabs fell off and left a scarred and pitted skin. Between 20 and 40 percent of those who caught the disease died. Those who survived were immune to future attacks.

Smallpox is rare today because of prevention through vaccination. This disfiguring disease was common, however, on the Western frontier and had no effective treatment. Smallpox frequently ravaged frontier communities, leaving the survivors with scars on their faces and bodies. Interestingly, this led to a different perception of beauty in the West than exists today. Many otherwise plain women were considered to be beautiful merely because they had smooth skin that had not been ravaged by smallpox. The pitting and scarring of smallpox on men's faces has been theorized to have been partially responsible for the popularity of full, bushy beards.

There was no specific treatment for smallpox, and approximately half the infected cases died. Advice for treating smallpox was to bathe the patient with cool water, or perhaps use a solution of lead acetate in a poultice. Mercury, in ointment form, was used to reduce contact with supposed noxious air and prevent the blisters of smallpox from developing. Because the cause of the disease was a virus, these "cures" were useless.

Attempts to control the spread of smallpox consisted of identification of disease cases, isolation of infected individuals, and vaccination of the rest of the local population. The infected were often quarantined in cabins, shacks, or tents outside town limits in what were termed "smallpox hospitals," but which were, in reality, pesthouses for contagious diseases.

After the arrival of the white man on the frontier, smallpox continually ravaged Indian tribes. An epidemic among the Pawnee killed off almost half the tribe in 1831. A particularly severe epidemic was inadvertently started among the Indians of the Great Plains in 1837 when an infected blanket was stolen from a steamboat. By the time the disease had run its course, an estimated 15,000 Plains Indians, including Mandan, Crow, and Blackfeet, had perished.

Epidemics broke out among the Comanche in 1839 and 1840. In 1854, smallpox infected the Utes. By 1855, the Arapaho were decimated by smallpox and other white man's diseases, such as erysipelas, whooping cough, and diarrhea. They were also plagued by venereal disease and alcoholism. In 1861, smallpox struck the Comanche again. In 1862, another severe epidemic of smallpox broke out among the Cheyenne and other Plains Indians, including a repeat for the Comanche. This epidemic was so bad that in 1863 the government sent a doctor to vaccinate the Arapaho against the disease. In 1883 smallpox again ravaged the Ute.

Smallpox also spread rapidly among white settlers. Deadwood, South Dakota, was hit hard by an epidemic of the disease in 1876. Between 1876 and 1878, widespread outbreaks of scarlet fever, diphtheria, and smallpox took the lives of many of Deadwood's children. Silver City, New Mexico, was similarly ravaged in 1877.

One of the legendary smallpox stories in the West concerned a dance-hall girl named Silverheels. She arrived in the mining town of Buckskin Joe in central Colorado in 1860 or 1861 and was immediately nicknamed for the silver-heeled slippers that she liked to wear. She was well-known and well-liked in the community.

In 1861, smallpox struck the small town, possibly brought by Mexican sheepherders who were passing through the area. Mines, businesses, and dance halls closed. Silverheels, temporarily out of a job, turned to nursing sick miners. She fixed their food, washed their clothing, and cleaned their cabins. With all this close exposure to the disease, she eventually caught it.

Before the disease ran its course, over 1,800 miners died. After the epidemic had passed, the grateful miners tried to find Silverheels to give her their thanks. But, apparently, she had quietly left town, probably because she thought that she could no longer ply her previous profession with a pockmarked face. The miners, unable to personally thank her, instead gave the name Mount Silverheels to a beautiful mountain nearby.

Years later there were reports of a veiled woman who appeared in the cemetery at Buckskin Joe and left flowers on the graves of miners who had died of smallpox. Some said it was Silverheels wearing a veil to hide her

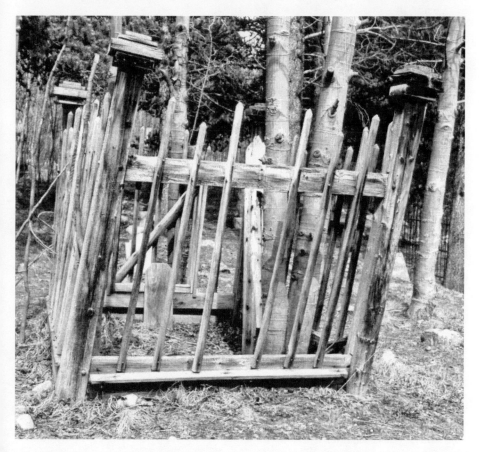

When the gold ran out, the tiny town of Buckskin Joe in Colorado was abandoned by all but the ghosts of the smallpox victims buried in this cemetery (author's collection).

disfigured face. Nobody ever found out if it was her or not. It has been said that the ghost of Silverheels still roams the cemetery today.

Vaccination

Attempts to prevent smallpox went back as far as the sixteenth century and early forms of inoculation. The procedure was basically to open one of the smallpox blisters on a victim with a toothpick (a knife might have scared the victim) and introduce the clear serum from inside into a small scratch or puncture wound in the skin of the person being inoculated. This procedure was called "variolation," after one name for the disease. The patient being inoculated almost always became ill with smallpox.

Inoculation by this method usually produced a milder attack of the disease than the victim would have had from catching it spontaneously, and it did provide protection against future attacks of smallpox. However, this was a dangerous and uncertain method. There were the risks of other infection from the procedure, and the virulence of the smallpox being introduced was unknown. A few patients received no protection, while others contracted a violent case of the disease and died. A much safer procedure was vaccination, which introduced a limited amount of virus that had been produced under controlled conditions.

Physician Edward Jenner in England is usually credited with the discovery of vaccination for smallpox by using inoculation with cowpox. Cowpox was a different and less severe strain of the disease, but it also produced immunity against smallpox. Several others researchers may have experimented with cowpox before Jenner, but he was the one who reduced the procedure to successful practice and has been given the credit.

Though successful vaccination was developed by Jenner in 1796, the practice was not widespread for a long time afterwards. As a result, any smallpox outbreak was a serious threat to those who came into contact with it.

Tuberculosis

Tuberculosis, or TB for short, was the scourge of nineteenth century America. The disease was more commonly known in Victorian times as "consumption" or the "White Plague." The bacterium that caused it is one of the oldest disease agents known to man and has probably been infecting humans for over 10,000 years. Tuberculosis was widespread in the second half of the nineteenth century as a result of poor nutrition and crowded living conditions. The disease was contracted by inhaling bacteria-laden air or by swallowing the bacterium in food or drink, particularly in milk from an infected cow. Direct contact, such as kissing, also transmitted the disease. Tuberculosis spread rapidly throughout the Old West, and was particularly common at the high altitudes encountered by many prospectors and miners in the Rocky Mountain West.

The cause of tuberculosis was the bacillus *Mycobacterium tuberculosis*, which was spread by droplets from an infected person's cough. Consequently, the common frontier practice of spitting in public, such as on the floor in saloons, was a serious health problem.

Tuberculosis could infect many parts of the body, but typically attacked the lungs. The reason that it was called the "White Plague" was that, as the disease progressed, the bacteria caused destruction of lung tissue and the lungs filled with white, spongy material. Eventually the victims suffered massive lung hemorrhage and death. Other symptoms were fever, night sweats, a bloody cough, and weight loss. Because tuberculosis primarily affected the lungs, victims were known as "lungers."

The cause of tuberculosis was not known to early physicians in the West. Physician Arthur Hertzler recalled "a young girl who, following baptism by immersion, died a few months later of galloping consumption. The scoffers attributed the tuberculosis to the exposure."[10]

Even in the early 1880s, tuberculosis was still thought to be caused by some combination of poor diet, dissolute lifestyle, harsh climate, and poor mental state. It wasn't until 1882 that Robert Koch showed that the true cause was a bacillus. However, as late as 1893 a paper published in the *Journal of the American Medical Association* hypothesized that tuberculosis was a nervous disease.[11]

Until the true cause of the disease was discovered, various early medical therapies were tried and proven ineffective. Dubious treatments included drinking kerosene, creosote, or copious amounts of whiskey. In an alternative therapy, tuberculosis was thought to be cured by the pure, fresh air of the mountains of the West. As a result, Colorado, Arizona, New Mexico, and California attracted many of those who had contracted the disease. Colorado was such a popular destination that it received the nickname of the "World's Sanitarium." Indeed, "lungers" did seem to improve with the higher altitude and a regimen of outdoor living, eating healthy food and enjoying rest, fresh air, sunshine, and exercise. The improvement was probably due to these factors boosting the victim's immune system, which helped to at least slow the worsening of the disease.

Fresh air was an important part of the treatment, and those with the disease slept in open, unheated, outside porches and lived in tent camps in all weather. Sometimes tuberculosis patients felt so much better in the high dry climate of the West that they thought they were cured. Some left the beneficial

climate and went back home, where they went into a relapse and dropped
dead.

One of the best-known sufferers of tuberculosis in the Old West was
John Henry "Doc" Holliday, one of the participants in the Gunfight at the
OK Corral that took place in Tombstone, Arizona, on October 26, 1881. Holliday contracted tuberculosis in 1871 after attending dental school in Baltimore. In line with the thinking at the time, doctors recommended that he
travel to the West, to Colorado or Arizona, for his health. Holliday led an
active life, playing cards professionally and gambling his way around the Old
West. He finally succumbed to his disease on November 8, 1887. He died at
the Hotel Glenwood in Glenwood Springs, Colorado, and was buried in
nearby Linwood Cemetery in a grave that has not been definitely located to
this day.

One of only three facilities in the country dedicated to the research and
treatment of tuberculosis was Fort Bayaud near present-day Silver City, New

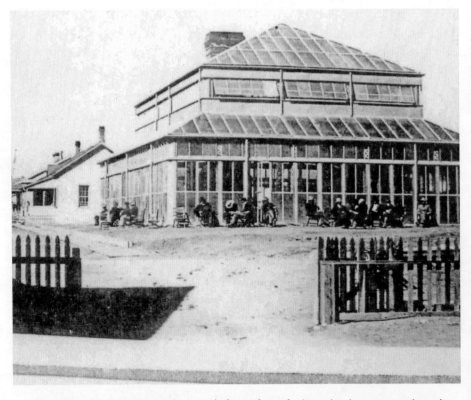

Fort Bayard, New Mexico, the army's first tuberculosis sanitarium, put patients in
this large solarium to allow consumption victims exposure to sunlight (thought
to be a large part of the cure) year round (author's collection).

Mexico. The fort was originally built as a military outpost in reaction to the Indian Wars of the Southwest during the latter half of the nineteenth century. After the Indians were placed on the reservation, troops were no longer needed at the fort. The high altitude and dry climate made it the ideal location for tuberculosis sufferers, and in 1899 the fort was transferred to the Army Medical Department to become the army's first TB sanitarium. Doctors from around the country came to the fort to learn the latest treatments for the disease. A large solarium allowed soldiers with TB to be exposed to sunlight year round.

Typhoid

Typhoid, also known as "malignant bilious fever" or "slow fever," was another of the horrible diseases prevalent in the Old West. The mortality rate for those who contracted it was anywhere from 25 to 56 percent.

Typhoid fever was the result of a severe infection caused by the bacterium *Salmonella typhosa* (now known as *Salmonella typhi*), which was not identified until 1880 by Karl Eberth and Georg Gaffky. Man is the only species susceptible to typhoid, and humans act as carriers. In the 1890s, between 300,000 and 400,000 cases were reported in the United States.

Transmission of typhoid was through improperly prepared food or milk, and particularly through contact with contaminated water supplies. Even dishes or food washed in contaminated water could spread the disease. The disease was therefore commonly transmitted on the Oregon and Santa Fe Trails through springs and water holes that occurred in low spots where human waste drained. In many instances, it came from contamination of water supplies that occurred when privies were placed too close to wells. Another source of transmission of typhoid were common houseflies that came in contact with feces containing bacteria and carried the disease to food or water.

Symptoms of typhoid include a rising temperature, followed by high fever, a skin rash, abdominal pain, and diarrhea. The bacterium damaged the lining of the small intestine. As a consequence, the victims died from internal bleeding and dehydration, or from blood poisoning. Patients became severely ill for several weeks. Recovery, if it was going to take place, happened at about the third week; however, patients could suffer for as long as a month before dying.

The symptoms of cholera and typhoid were similar, and it was not until 1880 that the difference between the two could be routinely diagnosed. Typhoid symptoms were also similar to those of malaria, thus leading to further confusion in reaching a correct diagnosis. Early physicians incorrectly believed that catching typhoid was the result of unfortunate heredity, a predisposition towards the disease, or to unknown factors in the environment.

Early doctors prescribed purging and enemas for both diseases, which was exactly the wrong thing to do—the increase in dehydration caused by these treatments was the opposite of what was required, which was re-hydration with fluids. A decrease of approximately 7 percent of water in the body is enough to shut down circulation of the blood and cause death.

Not all the people who carried typhoid bacteria within them became ill, but they could still transmit the disease to others. The bacterium was carried in the gall bladder and intestines of these human carriers and was excreted in their feces and urine. Two to 3 percent of people infected with typhoid were carriers who had no obvious symptoms. The spread of disease by healthy human carriers was not unusual, and carriers also existed for diphtheria, dysentery, cholera, and meningitis.

The best-known example of a typhoid carrier was Mary Mallon, who became famous as "Typhoid Mary" because she transmitted the disease to others without becoming ill herself. She was a reservoir for typhoid while she worked as a cook in various cities in the Northeast in the early 1900s. Though apparently immune herself, she spread the disease wherever she cooked. She was tracked down in 1907 and institutionalized in Riverside Hospital on Long Island after she attacked doctor George Soper with a meat cleaver. She was released in 1910 under the promise that she would give up cooking. In spite of the promise, however, she continued preparing meals and, after more deaths associated with her cooking, was sentenced to quarantine for life at Riverside Hospital, where she died twenty-eight years later.

An effective test for typhoid was not developed until 1896, with Fernand Widal's agglutination test for antibodies in the blood. Today, treatment for the disease is with antibiotics, and vaccination is available for prevention.

Typhus

Typhus, not to be confused with typhoid, was an inclusive name for any one of several acute infectious diseases, such as trench fever, epidemic typhus, and relapsing fever. Typhus was also known as "hospital fever," "ship fever," and "jail fever" because those were places with concentrated populations of people where the disease was commonly found. Typhus was transmitted from human to human by *Rickettsia* (a microorganism occupying a position in size between bacteria and viruses) carried by body lice and bedbugs. In one form the disease was transmitted by fleas.

Typhus was characterized by blotchy, purplish spots on the body (which also gave it the name of "spotted fever"), peeling skin, loss of sight, and falling hair. As the disease progressed, the victim became disabled by chills, fever, listlessness, headache, and pain. An eventual downhill progression led to delirium, convulsions, coma, and perhaps death, which could occur in as high as 20 percent of the infected victims.

Recognizing these neurological symptoms, the name "typhus" was derived from a Greek word that meant "stupor." Because of the inability of doctors to differentiate between various infectious diseases, typhus was often considered to be the same as typhoid, though the two could be differentiated by the spots on the chest and abdomen that occurred with typhus.

Typhus occurred frequently in the crowded unsanitary conditions of an army camp or battlefield. It has been a common soldier's disease throughout the ages and has been severe enough in combat situations that its occurrence on one side or the other may have influenced the course of history.[12]

Yellow Fever

Yellow fever was mostly a disease of the South, but it also broke out in the California gold fields, carried there by Forty-Niners who crossed the Isthmus of Panama on their way to the mining camps. The disease was spread by the female *Aedes aegypti* mosquito, but it was not until 1901 that the mosquito's role was conclusively proven.

Yellow fever, also known as "Great Sickness," "American Plague," "Yellow Jack," or "Bilious Plague," arrived in the United States from Africa, via the West Indies, in slave and cargo ships, then flourished in puddles and rain barrels in southern seaports. Symptoms, which lasted about a week, included fever, vomiting, pain in the head and back, and skin which eventually developed the yellow color of jaundice (hence the name yellow fever), demonstrating the involvement of the liver. Between 20 and 50 percent of those who caught the disease eventually died.

Several yellow fever epidemics occurred in the East and South in the late 1700s and 1800s. In 1762, a severe epidemic of yellow fever broke out in Philadelphia. In attempts to ward off the disease, heated vinegar was sprinkled on the walls of buildings. This preventative may have had some merit, as the hot vinegar fumes may have driven mosquitoes out of the houses. Tobacco was also thought to prevent the disease, and even women and children went around smoking cigars. Again, the smoke may have had some beneficial effects by helping keep away disease-carrying mosquitoes. Camphor impregnated into a handkerchief and held to the mouth may have provided the same benefit. In desperation, people chewed garlic and inhaled camphor fumes. Other attempts to ward off the disease included lighting fires (which may have created dense smoke and dispersed the mosquitoes) and shooting off cannons to "agitate" the air.[13]

During the 1792 Philadelphia epidemic, and again in 1793, one of the foremost physicians to treat the disease was Benjamin Rush. Rush's cure for yellow fever was based on a combination of extensive bleeding and purging with calomel. His "cure" was not successful. Rush's sister and three of his five apprentices died from the disease. Rush did note that those who lived in smoky houses often escaped the disease but did not make the connection that smoke kept away mosquitoes. The real problem, of course, was that Philadelphia at the time had no sewage system or sanitary water supply, so that sewage festering in the streets and standing water attracted mosquitoes.

Yellow fever was initially not a major problem in the Western states, and it was mostly found in Southern seaports and towns. New Orleans experienced epidemics in 1853, 1854, 1855, 1858, 1867, and with similar regularity until 1905, when understanding of the role of the mosquito allowed prevention measures.

Forty-Niners rushing to the California gold fields commonly picked up yellow fever in Panama in Chagres, where mosquitoes swarmed along the Chagres River, and took it with them. In 1849, the fastest way to California from the East was by sea. One route consisted of making a five to eight month voyage in a sailing ship down the east side of South America, around Cape Horn and its unpredictable weather, and up the west side of the South American continent to San Francisco, for a mammoth journey of about 13,000 miles.

The other choice for sea travel was to sail from New York or Boston to the village of Chagres on the Atlantic side of the Isthmus of Panama. Once there, the traveler had to find some way to complete sixty overland miles to Panama City and hope to catch a ship that was headed north to the goldfields.

The Panama route could theoretically be traveled in less than two months. Unfortunately, many found that the jungle crossing took far longer than that. Yellow fever was endemic in Panama, and travelers contracted it while crossing the Isthmus. Hundreds of travelers fell ill with fever, and many died from other illnesses and accidental encounters with the alligators and poisonous snakes that infested the jungle. Constant hazards to contend with on the way were malaria, cholera, and yellow fever, along with an ominous-sounding affliction called "fermentation of the bowels." The incubation period for yellow fever, here also called "Panama fever," was about a week; therefore, someone who contracted the disease in Panama City wouldn't know about it until he was well on his way to the California gold fields. Once the Forty-Niners were on a ship, they found that they had not escaped from disease, as shipboard epidemics of measles and yellow fever were common.

Other Diseases

Other miscellaneous diseases plagued the Western settler. The organisms that transmitted tetanus (lockjaw) were common in the soil and could be absorbed through a simple cut or via an open arrow or gunshot wound sustained during a fight. As the name implies, the classic symptom was stiffness of the jaw, which then developed into muscular spasms that contorted the body to the point that the victim could not swallow or breathe. The patient died either from asphyxiation or from exhaustion due to the constant muscle spasms.

Botulism, caused by a deadly toxin produced by the organism *Clostridium botulinum*, was a danger that always lurked in improperly cooked or preserved food. The organism was found in the soil and in the intestinal tract of domestic animals. Contamination of preserved food during home canning could cause death through paralysis of the heart and breathing.

Rocky Mountain spotted fever, also known as "black measles," was a disease spread by the bite of a wood tick, which transmitted the bacterium *Rickettsia ricketsii*. The disease could attack mountain men, cowboys, miners, loggers, and anyone who worked or spent much time in the outdoors. Occurring mostly in the Rocky Mountains, the Sierra Nevada Mountains, and the wooded area of the Pacific coast, the disease was debilitating though not usually fatal.

A less-common but very serious disease in the Old West was dengue (pronounced "den-gay") fever, which was a viral disease transmitted by the same *Aedes aegypti* mosquito that transmitted yellow fever. As did yellow fever, this disease came to the United States from the West Indies. During the course of the disease the victim suffered from excruciating pain in the back, hips, and extremities. The name dengue was a West Indian or Spanish corruption of the words "dandy fever," which described the dandified way of walking caused by the severe leg pains that accompanied the disease. Severe muscle spasms that racked the victims occasionally resulted in broken bones, giving it the alternate name of "breakbone fever." Like yellow fever, there was no cure, and about 5 percent of those who caught the disease died from it.

Other strange, vague "fevers" plagued settlers in the Old West. In the Rocky Mountain gold camps, and also in mining camps in the Sierras, miners and prospectors suffered from a mysterious disease called "mountain fever." The symptoms were high fever, aching bones and muscles, and painful headaches. The cause of the disease was never explained. The symptoms have been theorized to have been a type of Rocky Mountain tick fever, or possibly a form of typhoid. Another theory was that these symptoms were a type of altitude sickness because they only occurred at high altitudes.

A less common disease was erysipelas, which resulted in a high fever and hot, swollen skin. This occurred primarily in winter and, in line with the miasmatic theories, was consequently thought to be due to some taint in warm indoor air. Actually, it was caused by *Streptococcus* bacteria, which caused swelling in the tissue underneath the skin. Like other streptococcal diseases, it was highly contagious, and both doctors and nurses frequently caught it from dealing with patients with skin disorders.

Diabetes, which is estimated to afflict approximately 7 percent of today's population, was rare in the Old West. The reason was probably that foods in the Old West were not rich in sugar and processed fats, as are today's fast food meals. Doctors on the frontier were able to diagnose *diabetes mellitus* by tasting a small drop of the patient's urine, which had a sweet taste of honey.

CHAPTER FIVE

Unmentionable Diseases

One series of diseases that were not as frequently discussed in the Old West as other communicable diseases were the venereal diseases, a general category that included a multitude of sexually-transmitted diseases. Catching a venereal disease was referred to in the vernacular of the Old West as "being burned."

The most common venereal diseases were syphilis and gonorrhea. The organisms that caused them were fragile and did not live long outside the human body; therefore, they were primarily transmitted by direct sexual contact. Early physicians, believing that venereal disease was caused by excessive indulgence in sex, adapted the name "venereal" from the name Venus, the Roman goddess of love.

Venereal disease was rampant in the Old West in the second half of the nineteenth century, but Victorian attitudes made those who contracted it reluctant to discuss such personal health issues. Single men were the primary carriers of venereal disease, and they passed it back and forth during contact with prostitutes. However, it was not unusual for a respectable Victorian married woman to catch a venereal disease from her husband, who had picked it up while visiting a prostitute.

Victorian attitudes towards sex were a combination of prudery, repression, and obsession, making anything to do with sexual activities, particularly diseases that were often contracted through illicit relations, a subject that was taboo for polite conversation. This reticence led to a lack of knowledge about sexual matters, and misinformation was widespread. Due to a lack of understanding of the biological processes that were the basis for procreation, for example, one incorrect pronouncement found in some medical manuals of the time was that the "safe" time for having sex without pregnancy was precisely at the time in a woman's cycle when conception was most likely to occur. Another was that male orgasms were thought to weaken men, cause physical deterioration, and lead to retarded intellectual development.

Physicians felt that women, in particular, should not have sexual urges

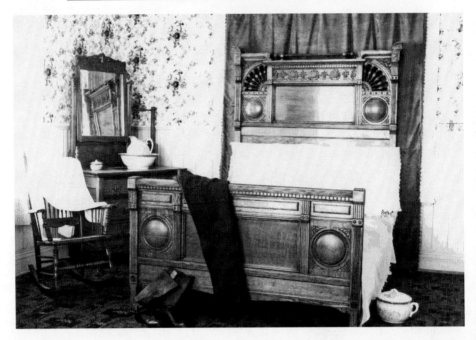

Here is where it all started for many men. Venereal disease was commonly transmitted via the bedroom of a brothel, both from prostitute to customer and vice versa. The washbasin on the stand was for washing before and afterwards, and the chamber pot on the floor was for other needs (Glenn Kinnaman, Colorado and Western History Collection).

or experience any enjoyment from sex, and that excessive sexual activity led to mental exhaustion and disorders of the reproductive organs.[1] Female orgasms, called "voluptuous spasms," were thought to interfere with conception and, if experienced often enough, would lead to sterility. Orgasms in women were also thought to induce unnatural passions for pepper, mustard, and cloves. A further perverse idea was that the enjoyment of sexual excitement in women was thought to be a symptom of impending insanity. To take this idea one step further, the insatiable sexual appetites of nymphomania were considered to be a type of madness and sufficient reason to be incarcerated in a mental asylum.

Venereal disease first appeared in the West via early fur trappers and traders who formed sexual liaisons with friendly Indian women. The native women, in turn, took the disease back to the men of their tribes. A second wave of venereal disease spread rapidly throughout the West after the Civil War, carried by ex-soldiers from the northern and southern armies, and by soldiers fighting in the Indian Wars. Estimates were that 38 percent of the soldiers fighting in the Civil War had venereal disease. In 1875, the U.S. Army reported 2,626 active cases of venereal disease. Some of the figures are difficult to interpret with precision because army surgeons did not distinguish between syphilis and gonorrhea, and lumped them both together for the purposes of reporting and treatment. At some frontier posts, the figure was estimated to be as high as 60 percent. In 1893, the U.S. Army Medical Corps estimated the overall incidence of venereal disease in frontier troops to be a little over 7 percent.

Venereal disease was further spread by cowboys, prospectors, and the host of settlers and gold miners who colonized the West. Prostitutes and their customers were responsible for the majority of the spread of venereal diseases. Contemporary estimates were that 50 percent of the prostitutes in the Old West had syphilis. Most prostitutes douched with antiseptic to try to prevent catching a venereal disease, but some did not consider this to be an essential practice, particularly on a busy night with many customers, or if the woman had been drinking heavily or using narcotic drugs. Prostitutes used strong antiseptic solutions, such as bichloride of mercury, mercuric cyanide, potassium permanganate, or carbolic acid. With frequent use, these harsh chemical solutions created internal irritation and general physical discomfort. Furthermore, douching was not always a sufficient safeguard against disease.

A prostitute usually inspected and washed off her customer with soap

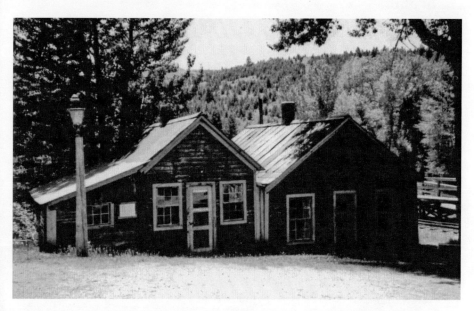

Brothels and their inmates were found in towns and cities throughout the West. These two adjoining wooden buildings made up the Green Front Boarding House bordello in Virginia City, Montana (author's collection).

and water, or carbolic acid, as a safeguard before sex, to prevent catching a venereal disease from him. She might wash him off afterwards to prevent him claiming that he had caught a disease from her. Another method was to use an antiseptic salve, such as boric acid mixed in petroleum jelly. Experienced prostitutes squeezed the base of the man's penis to determine if he had any discharge that would indicate the presence of gonorrhea. She might also stall for fifteen minutes or so before having sex with him to make sure that there was no further evidence of discharge.

Because venereal disease was rarely discussed, contemporary hospital records rarely listed venereal disease as a cause of death, but might put the cause down to "cancer of the brain" or some other vague term. This diagnosis did have some validity, however, because some of the inmates of mental asylums were those who had contracted syphilis earlier, and it had advanced into the late stage and destroyed the brain. In 1875, for example, Dr. C.C. Green from Virginia City, Nevada, was sent to an insane asylum in Woodbridge, California, with marked symptoms of mental decay. His work included treating prostitutes from the red light district in Virginia City, and apparently he caught one of their venereal diseases, probably syphilis.

Syphilis

The origins of syphilis have not been clearly identified, though there is evidence that syphilis existed in American Indians at least 500 years before the arrival of white explorers from the Old World. Further evidence supports two different theories. One, named the "Columbian Theory," is that syphilis originated in the Americas, and that Columbus and the Spanish soldiers who accompanied him picked up the disease in 1493 through contact with native women and carried it back to Europe with them. The other theory, named the "Environmental Theory," was that syphilis was a mutation of the tropical disease treponematosis that originated in tropical Africa. It appeared to be the same as several subspecies that caused the diseases yaws and pinta, both of which were disabling tropical afflictions.

The first theory makes possible historical sense, as Europe's first epidemic of syphilis broke out in 1495 during a conflict between the Spanish and the French. French troops had laid siege to the city of Naples, which was being defended by Spanish mercenaries who were though to have brought the disease with them. The syphilis-riddled army was finally forced by disease to return home to France, carrying the seeds of pestilence with them.

In 1530, an Italian physician, Girolamo Fracastoro (also known as Fracatorius), wrote a poem in Latin titled "Syphilis, Sive Morbus Gallicus," which was translated as "Syphilis, or the French Disease." It was the story of a shepherd named Sifilo, who had symptoms that characterized the disease. From that time on, "syphilis" was the usual name.

Syphilis was also called "the French Pox," or "the French Disease," because it was believed to have originated in France. However, everybody blamed somebody else. The French, who believed that it came from Italy, called it "the Neapolitan Disease." In Naples it was "the French Disease," and the English called it "the Spanish Disease." In Europe, syphilis was originally called "the Great Pox" because of the characteristic rash that accompanied the early stages of the infection and to distinguish it from the "small pox" (later spelled in one word, as smallpox). In the Old West, syphilis was typically referred to as just "the pox." It was also known as "lues," which was a general name for any pestilence or plague, but particularly syphilis. More colorful nicknames for the disease in the Old West were "old dog," "old ral," and "gambler's rot."

Syphilis progressed through several stages. Symptoms of the primary stage typically appeared from two weeks to three months after sex with an infected person. The tell-tale symptom was the eruption of a chancre, an ulcer-like sore on the skin shaped like a little crater, at the site of the entry of the bacteria into the body. This was typically on or around the external genitals. If untreated, the chancre went away by itself within two to ten weeks after it appeared. In reality, the external symptoms disappeared but the disease itself had not gone away.

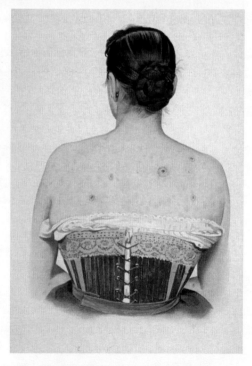

The secondary stage of syphilis manifested from one to six months after the chancre first appeared, when a generalized rash appeared on the body. A distinguishing feature of this stage was that the coppery-red rash did not hurt or itch. The rash was sometimes accompanied by other symptoms, such as a sore throat, headaches, joint pain, and a low-grade fever. Without treatment, these symptoms went away spontaneously in two to six weeks. At this point the disease

Nasty-looking sores that showed up all over the body were part of the symptoms of the secondary stage of syphilis (National Library of Medicine).

entered the latent stage. There were no symptoms, but the unseen syphilis bacteria invaded the heart, the bones, and the nervous system. This latent stage could last for years— up to twenty-five to thirty — and, in about half of the infected people, never progressed any further.

The other half went into the tertiary, or late, stage. In this destructive stage of syphilis, symptoms re-occurred. Skin ulcers and abscesses appeared as the disease burrowed into the circulatory and nervous systems. There was degeneration of the muscles, heart, skin, bones, joints, digestive system, genitals, and lungs. This could occur as late as forty years after the initial infection with the disease. Deterioration of the nose was a characteristic symptom at this stage. The brain and spinal cord were often attacked, which led to insanity, paralysis, and death. About 25 percent of all untreated cases progressed to the dementia stage, resulting in transfer to an insane asylum.

Syphilis was the subject of much misinformation. As late as 1900, one authority stated that syphilis could be spread by wearing a tight-fitting hat, by licking the same envelope as another person, or by using a lead pencil and holding the point between the lips.[2] Other misinformation was that syphilis could be transmitted by using the same towel or soap as an infected person. The longest-lasting old wives tale from the late 1800s was that syphilis was spread via toilet seats. In fact, syphilis was typically spread by sexual contact. However, it was true that during the secondary stage, when the disease could produce eruptions inside the mouth, it could be transmitted via saliva by kissing if there was a break in the skin in or around the mouth of the uninfected person. The chances of catching syphilis from an infected sex partner have been estimated at between 30 and 50 percent. Men appear to be more susceptible to catching syphilis than women.

In 1905, Fritz Schaudinn and Erich Hoffman identified a bacterium that they named *Spirocheta pallida*, but which later received the modern name of *Treponema pallidum*. The bacterium took the shape of a spiral screw, hence it was called a spirochete.

An important breakthrough in identifying the disease occurred when August von Wasserman and his colleagues developed a diagnostic blood test for syphilis to identify those without symptoms. The test was named the Wasserman Test after him.

Gonorrhea

The other common venereal disease that spread rapidly over the Old West was gonorrhea, also called "the clap," "the drip," and "the gleet." It was the oldest of the sexually-transmitted diseases and has been described both in the Bible and in early Chinese writings.[3]

Physicians in the Old West estimated that between 50 and 80 percent of all men between the ages of eighteen and thirty contracted gonorrhea at some point in their lives. Contracting gonorrhea was not as serious as syphilis; nonetheless, it was a dangerous disease that could be accompanied by inflammation, fever, vomiting, and abdominal distress. In its worst cases it could produce serious eye infections, kidney damage, and disabling arthritis. Gonorrhea caused pain and occasional sterility, but syphilis often killed the infected person.

Some Western towns set up a process of inspection of prostitutes once a week to test and, if necessary, treat them for venereal disease. However, the incubation period for gonorrhea was only two to eight days after infection, thus increasing the probability of the rapid unknowing spread of disease to many customers.

The primary symptom of gonorrhea was a discharge from the genitals. Early physicians sometimes mistook the discharge for semen; hence, in 130 A.D. the Greek physician Galen gave it the modern name that means "morbid discharge of semen." The true cause was not discovered until 1879 when Albert Neisser identified the *Neisseria gonorrhoeae* bacterium. The bacteria were fragile and did not live long outside the body, and so had to be transmitted by direct sexual contact. Studies have shown that the risk of acquiring gonorrhea after sex with an infected person is about 30 percent.

In almost all men, gonorrhea produced infection of the urethra, which rapidly resulted in a purulent (pus-like) discharge. Though other forms of venereal disease produced a similar discharge, at the time they were all lumped together under the heading of "gonorrhea." The gonorrhea discharge was accompanied by a burning sensation when urinating and by swelling of the lymph nodes of the groin. Because these symptoms were obvious and painful, men tended to seek medical treatment right away. Without treatment, the pain became worse as the infection spread up the urinary tract and affected the prostate and bladder.

In women, the symptoms of gonorrhea were not so obvious, and in about 80 percent of females with gonorrhea there were no symptoms at all. If untreated, the disease invaded the uterus and the rest of the reproductive tract, and eventually caused sterility. The bacteria could spread to the joints, the eyes, or the heart, causing more serious problems. These women did not know that they were infected and, particularly in the case of prostitutes in cattle and mining towns of the Old West, who had frequent multiple sexual contacts, were likely to spread the disease before anyone knew where they had got it.[4]

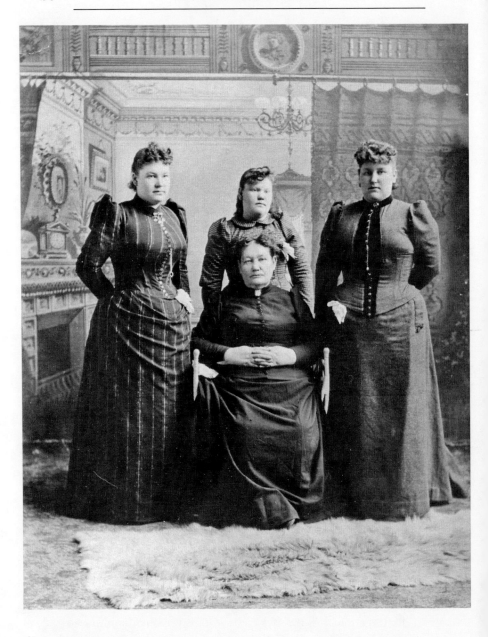

Prostitution was common all over the West in the late 1800s. Jane Elizabeth Ryan, seated in the middle, ran a bordello in the Market Street brothel district in Denver, Colorado. Daughters Julia, Mona, and Annie, standing around her, all worked there (copyright Colorado Historical Society; Mazzulla Collection, scan #10035946).

Treatments and Cures

The treatment of choice today for both syphilis and gonorrhea is one or several doses of penicillin. In the Old West of the late 1800s there was no penicillin, and the "cures" were less effective.

In the mid–1800s there was no positive cure for syphilis. However, after the secondary stage of syphilis, the symptoms went away spontaneously, often for years. For this reason, even the most outlandish cures appeared to work effectively, and the patients felt themselves cured. Treatment for gonorrhea ranged from warm baths, herbal medicine, and poultices of tobacco to the old heroic standby of bleeding.

In 1860, the average cost of a cure for syphilis or gonorrhea was between ten and twenty dollars, but could be as high as a hundred dollars. Usually payment was demanded in advance of treatment. Doctors who frequently treated syphilis patients were derisively called "pox doctors."

Some doctors felt that the best treatment was to cauterize the genital sores with a red-hot iron. Unsympathetic doctors felt that the pain of this cure was the patient's reward for moral transgression. "Cures" were sometimes even more drastic. Dr. Hiller in Virginia City, Nevada, treated a thirty-five-year-old miner whose genitals were ravaged by the horrible sores that accompanied syphilis. His solution was to perform surgery and cut two inches from the unfortunate man's penis.

The standard cure for both syphilis and gonorrhea for many years was the "mercury cure." The common wry saying of the time was "A night with Venus; a lifetime with mercury." Mercury was given by mouth, as an ointment rubbed onto the skin, or administered by hypodermic injection. Red mercuric oxide was used as an ointment that was spread on syphilitic sores, and calomel (mercurous chloride) was taken by mouth. Mercury was also injected directly into the urethra with a piston syringe.

During the Lewis and Clark expedition, Lewis routinely treated the men with calomel pills. The expedition supplies included four penis syringes, so obviously the leaders expected to have to deal with frequent attacks of gonorrhea along the way. This number of syringes was apparently warranted because at least eight members of the expedition contracted venereal disease during the trip from friendly and willing Indian women from the Mandan, Shoshone, and Nez Percé tribes.

Mercury poisoning was always a risk in these treatments, and overdose led to excess salivation, loose teeth, bleeding gums, and various neurological problems that could result in insanity. After frequent or prolonged treatments, patients inevitably lost their teeth and developed sores in their mouths. The caution in one nursing text read: "[Mercury] is given until there is slight soreness of the gums and then the dose is reduced about half until these symptoms disappear." The mercury cure was not quick and easy, as the text continues: "The administration of mercury in some form should be continued for at least two-and-a-half years."[5]

Those who did not want to undergo the mercury cure could try a herbal medicine made from the wild iris plant (also known as blue flag). An alternative treatment was the use of Mormon tea, which was also called whorehouse tea but more politely desert tea. This practice was supposedly started by a Jack Mormon, who frequented a bordello named Katie's Place in Elko, Nevada, during the mining rush. Because of its supposed reputation for curing syphilis, Mormon tea became a standard fixture in brothels all over Nevada and California.

Another conventional medical treatment for the time was repeated irrigation of the urethra with a solution of lead acetate (also known as *saccharum saturni* or Goulard's powder) with a special penis syringe. Many men were too embarrassed to go through such a course of treatment, and so they waited and hoped that the symptoms would go away by themselves.

By the early 1900s a more advanced — and effective — cure for syphilis was available. In 1910, the mercury cure was replaced by the use of Salvarsan 606, an arsenic-based preparation that was injected directly into the body.[6] It was prepared as a yellow powder that was dissolved in water and given intravenously. Salvarsan was developed by the Nobel prize–winning German medical scientist Paul Ehrlich. He named the compound Salvarsan 606 because it was the six hundred and sixth preparation that he had tried. It was nicknamed "the magic bullet," and, indeed, its results were almost magical. Within three years Salvarsan had cured over 10,000 sufferers of syphilis. It was not without its drawbacks, however. The treatment was expensive, painful, and sometimes had severe side effects. It was difficult to administer and required a course of twenty to forty injections over a year's period. One of the unpleasant and possible serious side effects was a severe, itchy rash. It was, however, an effective and lasting cure. Salvarsan became the standard treatment for syphilis until 1945 and the widespread use of the antibiotic penicillin.

Not everybody was happy with Ehrlich's Salvarsan, however. Victorian moral reformers attacked his discovery on the grounds that it would encourage sexual relations. They felt that if Americans were going to sin, they should have to pay the price and accept the risks of catching a disease.

Patent medicines were also popular as self-proclaimed, sure-fire cures for venereal disease because they could be surreptitiously ordered over-the-counter at drugstores or anonymously via the mail. Popular patent medicines for venereal disease were Red Drops, Bumstead's Gleet Cure, and the Unfortunate's Friend. Pabst's Okay Specific advertised that it cured gonorrhea "positively and without fail ... no matter how serious or of how long standing." Another, available in liquor stores, was Pine Knot Bitters. One folk remedy for gonorrhea was to take pills made with turpentine three times a day. Whether this was effective or not was not recorded.

Contraception and Abortion

The result of sex for most Victorian women was pregnancy. If a woman wanted children, she would have to endure the pain and possible complications of childbirth, in those days called "confinement." Unless she were in perfect health, she literally risked her life to have the child because the chances of infection and a woman dying during childbirth were high. Breech birth or heavy bleeding could be fatal on an isolated ranch with no proper medical care at hand. Though some methods of contraception were known, and advertisements for them appeared in newspapers in big cities, they were mostly considered to be disagreeable and were generally unreliable.

Contraceptives

In the Victorian era, contraception was viewed as a method of separating sex from procreation and a way in which men could satisfy their supposedly continual lusts without having children. For this reason, birth control was generally viewed with disfavor, which was reflected in the large number of children — perhaps a dozen or more — in a typical family. The "correct" Victorian way to limit family size was by abstinence.

Several methods of contraception were considered to be reliable in the mid–1800s. One was the withdrawal method, where the man withdrew before orgasm. Though this was a popular method among married couples, it was unreliable. The man had to have enough control that he could stop before orgasm, even though his body told him to proceed. It was also unreliable because many men leaked sperm even before ejaculation.

Another method was the vaginal sponge, a small piece of sponge that was placed in the vagina before intercourse to block sperm. The sponge was typically soaked in lemon juice or quinine before use in an attempt to increase its effectiveness. Lemon juice, which naturally contained citric acid, was partially effective, as it could immobilize sperm. Quinine was thought to have contraceptive properties but was later found to be generally ineffective.

Other devices were used to block sperm. European immigrants brought with them the use of a primitive type of cervical cap that was made from bee's wax. An early design of diaphragm, named the "Wife's Protector," was patented in 1846 by J.B. Beers. The modern type of spring-loaded rubber diaphragm was described in 1882 by German physiologist C. Hasse, who wrote under the pseudonym of Wilhelm P.J. Mensinga. In 1883, Aletta Jacobs, a Dutch physician, described a similar diaphragm that was known as the "Dutch Cap."

The commonest method of contraception was the condom, often called "the sheath" or the "French Letter." The use of condoms was not totally reliable as a method of birth control and had a failure rate of about 10 percent. Early condoms were made from sheep's intestines. Rubber versions became available in the 1840s after Charles Goodyear developed a successful process for the vulcanization of India rubber. Condoms were commonly used by prostitutes to prevent transmission of venereal disease. This gave condoms an undesirable connotation and made their use unpopular among married couples as a method of limiting family growth.

The introduction of cured rubber in the 1840s also led to the development of rubber hygiene syringes, and douching became a widely used method of contraception. Various chemicals were used, including solutions of quinine, lemon juice, vinegar, alum, zinc sulfate, and iodine. Some of these chemicals were effective; most were not. The most popular chemical was car-

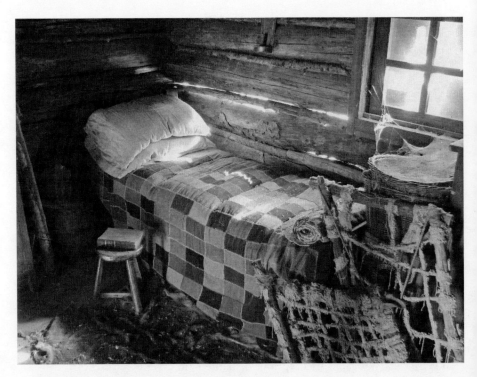

A drafty one-room log cabin on the frontier, with no running water or privacy, was certainly not an appealing place to practice contraception (author's collection).

bolic acid, the same strong antiseptic solution that was used by prostitutes in an attempt to guard against venereal disease.

Carbolic acid, also known as phenol, was a common disinfectant and could have other, more sinister uses. In March of 1921, Ann Hopkins walked into the Connor Hotel in the mining town of Jerome, Arizona, and threw a glass of carbolic acid into the face and eyes of Lucile Gallagher, whom she suspected of being her husband's mistress.

Though information about contraceptive methods was widespread and freely available at mid-century, in 1873 the distribution of devices and information on birth control became illegal and was punishable by law, when Congress passed an anti-obscenity bill called the "Comstock Act." The bill was named for Anthony Comstock, a self-appointed censor of American morals who persuaded Congress to pass a bill that included contraceptive devices and information as obscene material. Even doctors could be prosecuted for distributing contraceptive information to their patients. It was not until 1918 that physicians were again allowed to give birth control information to women who asked for it.

Many women in the rural West were isolated on ranches and farms, and the information they obtained was often by word of mouth from friends and neighbors—much of it incorrect. For many women who lived in log houses with no privacy, bathrooms or running water, contraceptive methods were not particularly appealing. As a result, many women relied on ineffective patent medicines that claimed to prevent pregnancy.

Abortions

Until the 1870s, the Victorian view of abortion and miscarriage was different than today. A woman determined for herself if she was pregnant, not the doctor, whom she probably did not see on a regular basis anyway, because babies were typically delivered at home with the help of a midwife. A woman decided that she was pregnant when the baby started moving, which was in about the fourth month. In nineteenth-century terminology this was called the "quickening." Before this happened, a woman might choose to consider herself pregnant or she might consider that she had an "unnatural blockage" or "unwanted obstruction" that was causing the cessation of menses, depending on whether she viewed the pregnancy as desirable or not.

Removing an "obstruction" was not considered a criminal offense, and she and her doctor felt justified in its removal (i.e., abortion) to restore regular menses. Typical of the "cures" was one in the 1852 version of the *Ladies' Indispensible Assistant*, which recommended taking a tablespoon of tincture of guaiacum in half a cup of milk at the full of the moon

Madame Costello, a female physician, openly advertised in a San Francisco newspaper that she could treat women for obstruction of their monthly periods. Dr. Bird advertised that she dispensed Dr. Vandenburgh's Female Renovating Pills, which were an effective remedy for "all cases where nature has stopped from any cause whatever."[7]

Abortions were considered to be immoral, but were performed using either surgical means or via drugs. Both methods were dangerous because of the lack of medical knowledge. Mechanical methods of abortion, which were also called an "illegal operation" or a "criminal operation," were particularly dangerous because of the risk of subsequent excessive bleeding or fatal infection. As with any surgical procedure of the time, severe illness or death from infection was the outcome in a high percentage of cases.

Drugs were employed to induce miscarriage, but their use involved a high risk of side effects. Ergot and quinine were two of the drugs used. Ergot, which was utilized by doctors to control excessive bleeding following childbirth, could be given in large doses to induce miscarriage. It was accompanied by toxic side effects that included vomiting, convulsions, blindness, severe abdominal cramps, and the development of gangrene in the fingers or toes. Alternatively, a massive dose of quinine could stimulate premature contractions. Again, the dose required to be effective in inducing miscarriage was so large that it exposed the woman to kidney damage, anemia, loosening of the teeth, and respiratory collapse.

Vigorous exercise, hot baths, deliberate falls down stairs, sustained horseback riding, douching with irritating or toxic chemicals, repeated large-volume enemas, or large doses of purgatives were also techniques employed to induce a miscarriage.

Miscarriages were sometimes deliberately induced by the wearing of tightly-laced corsets. The use of tight corsets allowed women to convince themselves that they had never really been pregnant in the first place and that the "obstruction" had finally cleared itself. Wearing tight corsets by pregnant women resulted in miscarriages, stillborn babies, malformed infants, and a high rate of mortality among fetuses that successfully survived to birth. Physician Alice Stockham wrote in 1883 that the direct cause of these problems was a lack of oxygen delivered to the fetus because constricting corsets inhibiting the mother's breathing. Stockham stated quite bluntly that "tight lacing [was] the chief cause of infant mortality."[8]

Another method was to use one of the many patent medicines advertised to relieve "obstructions," "blockage of monthly periods," or other vague terms. One such was Clark's Pills, which contained aloe, quinine, and ergot, among other ingredients. Another was Dr. Van Den Burgh's "female renovating pills."

Anti-abortion campaigns started in the 1850s and were aimed at making the use of a drug or mechanical means to induce a miscarriage a criminal offense. Efforts by doctors, religious leaders, and moral reformers culminated in laws in the 1870s that banned abortion. Home advice manuals for women, however, contained methods for the "removal of an obstruction" until the 1880s. Abortion continued to be performed, but it was outside the law.

Contemporary estimates indicate that perhaps 100,000 abortions were performed in the United States each year in the late 1800s. However, nobody really knew with any certainty, and this figure could only be a guess because the procedure was illegal and was only reported when the patient died.

CHAPTER SIX

Healing with Drugs

Heroic medicine to "rebalance" the humors was based in large part on drugs that achieved various effects on the patient's system. Chief among them were purgatives to cleanse the intestinal tract, drugs to induce vomiting, and various chemicals to induce sweating. The bowels, the mouth, and the pores of the skin were considered to be the main routes for driving noxious substances out of the body and restoring the balance of the humors.

Drugs on the early frontier were sometimes expensive due to a lack of supply. Everything in San Francisco, for example, during the rush of Forty-Niners was expensive. Flour sold for three to five dollars a pound, and a single apple might sell for two or three dollars. Even a common blanket might cost as much as forty dollars. In line with these exorbitant prices, many medicines were as much as ten dollars for a single dose. Laudanum sold for ten dollars a drop. One miner in California reportedly paid fifty dollars for enough laudanum to give him a good night's sleep.

In the mid–1800s, only a limited number of medications were available — or effective. The commonest ones were opium and morphine for controlling pain and treating dysentery, quinine to treat malaria, colchicine for gout, and mercury to "cure" syphilis. Drugs carried in a doctor's black bag typically included morphine, opium, calomel, Dover's powder, ammonia, quinine, and cathartic pills.

Purgatives

One of the cornerstones of heroic medicine involved purging the bowels to drive out "impure" humors that were causing an imbalance in the body and thus cleanse the system.[1] Purging was also thought to promote good health through purity of the bowels; neglect of the bowels was thought to send a person down the pathway to appalling disease.[2] One health writer even went so far as to propose that constipation would produce "congestion of the blood," which could lead to disturbed mental functioning. He contended that the resulting swollen blood vessels in the brain would send the sufferer into a downhill mental spiral and eventual life of crime, including robbery and murder.

The milder treatments in the purgative group involved laxative mineral salts. Typical were Glauber's salts (sodium sulfate) and Epsom salts (magnesium sulfate), both of which had a long history of use. Epsom salts were so effective that one poet in England in the 1650s penned the following couplet:

Some drink of it, and in an houre,
Their stomach, guts and kidneys scower.[3]

"Taking the waters" at fashionable spas in America or Europe that offered a course of treatment through drinking mineral waters (which often contained Epsom salts, Glauber's salts, Rochelle salts or some similar mineral salts) was a polite way of describing a series of violent purges. Extracts of various plants and roots, such as rhubarb or castor oil, were used to achieve the same results.

More powerful and dramatic purgatives included calomel, jalap, croton oil, and colocynth. Colocynth, delivered in the form of an enema, was recommended for kidney problems, paralysis, and palsy. Collectively these drugs were known as "physics," and their use was named "physicking."[4] Some purgative medicines produced such a series of profuse watery evacuations, and were accompanied by such severe intestinal cramping, that they were called "drastics."[5] One particularly powerful remedy was Plummer's pills, a combination of jalap, calomel, and antimony, each of which was a strong purgative when taken by itself.[6] Another powerful combination of purgatives was a combination of gamboge, aloes, rhubarb, castile soap, jalap, lobelia, and cayenne pepper in a molasses base. It was recommended in pill form for "billious [sic] and dyspeptic habits."

Croton oil was the main player in a somewhat humorous story reported from the army's Camp Crittenden in the Arizona Territory. A series of incidents occurred in which pies from the officer's mess "mysteriously" disappeared. Tiring of this, on the Fourth of July, 1869, the post surgeon added some croton oil to the next batch of pies. The pie thieves turned out to be two of the cooks. The two men became violently ill and called for the surgeon, as they thought they were having a bad attack of cholera. The doctor didn't have much sympathy and told them to stop eating so much pie. Needless to say, the pie-stealing stopped.

The use of these powerful purgatives was not for the faint of heart — or stomach. Croton oil was so strong that it could cause erosions of the mouth and esophagus. Colocynth was so active and such a violent purgative that in large doses it could cause nausea, vomiting, delirium, low blood pressure and sometimes death. It was eventually considered too dangerous to use as a drug and was withdrawn from medicinal use.

If a patient were unconscious, or for some other reason the oral route was impossible or difficult, clysters (enemas) of warm water were used to purge the system. Among the more peculiar enemas was one that contained boiled oatmeal gruel mixed with butter and salt.

Emetics

Another popular method to restore the humors by ridding the body of supposed impure substances that caused disease was to have the patient vomit them out. The use of emetic drugs was a popular treatment for "bilious attacks," dysentery, jaundice, and a variety of digestive problems. Vomiting was also induced in cases of bad water or tainted food, two of the few instances where the treatment was probably justified.

One of the most popular emetic drugs was tartar emetic, which was antimony and potassium tartarate. Other emetic drugs were ipecac, which was derived from plant roots, and honey dissolved in warm water. All of these emptied the stomach with predictable violence.

Sudorifics

A third method of expelling noxious substances from the body was thought to be to sweat them out. Medical theory stated that if the pores were clogged, waste matter, in the form of perspiration, was trapped inside the body where it would poison the individual from the inside.

Popular chemicals used to induce sweating were Dover's powder, camphor, and tartar emetic. Dover's powder was named after Dr. Thomas Dover, a British physician who developed his namesake medicine in 1732. His concoction consisted of one part opium and one part ipecac, mixed with lactose. The usual dosage in Dover's powder in the early 1900s was one grain of opium and one of ipecac. Dover claimed to have administered as much as ten grains of opium with ten grains of ipecac to patients in a single dose, or ten times as much of each ingredient. So powerful was this medicine, and so spectacular its result, that pharmacists who compounded Dover's original formula in the late 1700s often advised patients to make out their wills before taking the medicine.

One military surgeon on an expedition into the Black Hills of South Dakota during the Indian Wars included in his medical kit 1,200 opium pills,

1,200 quinine pills, 1,200 cathartic pills, and 10 pounds of Dover's powder. Medicinal whiskey and brandy were also part of every field medical kit.

As historian Stephen Ambrose noted, Lewis and Clark took with them "thirteen hundred doses of physic [purgatives], eleven hundred of emetic, thirty-five hundred of diaphoretic (sweat inducer) and more, including drugs for blistering, salivation, and increased kidney output, along with tourniquets, and clyster syringes."[7] Medical supplies also included fifteen pounds of Peruvian bark, half a pound of jalap, opium, six pounds of Glauber's salts, saltpeter (potassium nitrate, also called "niter"), two pounds of tartar emetic, laudanum, calomel, and mercury ointment. A powerful pharmacopoeia indeed.

Counter-Irritants

Counter-irritants were drugs intended to transfer irritation from a diseased area to another area by raising blisters on the skin. Blistering, for example, was used as a cure for pleurisy, which was irritation of the membranes surrounding the lungs. Some of the chemicals applied to the skin to cause blistering were mustard oil, turpentine, camphor, and gum ammoniac (the resin from a desert perennial plant from India). One surgical book of the era recommended that to produce an immediate and strong blistering response, boiling water should be poured directly onto the patient. The practice of counter-irritation largely stopped by the time of the Civil War.

Irritants were also given by mouth to act directly on the digestive tract, but they were so powerful that they often caused vomiting, pain, and shock.

A popular agent used for blistering was *cantharides*, also known as Spanish Fly. This medicine was made literally from the dried and powdered body of a bright green beetle (*Cantharis vesicatoria*) that was common in Spain, France, Italy, and Russia. The compound was spread on the skin in the form of a paste. Spanish Fly was also taken by mouth as a diuretic, and was used to treat paralysis, tetanus, and diabetes. It was also said to be successful for suppressing menstrual periods.

Spanish Fly was probably better-known and used as a reputed aphrodisiac. In reality, it was a powerful irritant of the urinary tract and genital system. It caused burning and painful urination that gave a sensation of continual stimulation of the genitals.

Heavy Metals

Several of the so-called "heavy metals," such as lead, arsenic, and mercury, were used as part of medical practice. These metals were extremely poisonous, thus making their use for drug therapy very dangerous.

Arsenic

Arsenic was a highly-toxic, tasteless metallic powder. It was so poisonous that it was used in weed killers and rat poison (it is also known as rat's bane). Various arsenic preparations, used medicinally in small doses, were prescribed for both internal and external conditions that varied from rheumatism to syphilis. Small doses of arsenic were thought to strengthen the lungs. It was also taken as a medicine by women to improve their complexions. Concocted as Fowler's solution, a weak solution of arsenic trioxide in water, arsenic was used to treat muscle twitching and pain caused by irritated nerves. Until the discovery of Salvarsan 606, arsenic was used as a treatment for syphilis.

For a short while, arsenic was thought to be a cure for the widespread curse of malaria, after some workmen in a copper smelting plant were found to be free from malaria. It was presumed that arsenic in the men's bodies was preventing the disease. After further investigation, however, doctors realized that arsenic fumes spreading freely throughout the factory had killed off the mosquitoes.

Mercury

The use of mercury and its compounds was widespread in nineteenth-century medicine. Bichloride of mercury was used as an antiseptic and was commonly employed by prostitutes as an antiseptic douche. Another use for the metal arose from the fact that mercury in oil held in the mouth produced intense salivation.

The commonest use for mercury was as calomel (mercurous chloride), which was widely utilized as a purge and a cure for what were considered to be "inflammatory diseases," such as cholera, typhoid, and fever from undetermined causes. Gastric problems, ranging from constipation to diarrhea, were treated with calomel. The advice given by old time doctors was: "When in doubt, give calomel."[8]

Calomel came in a large blue lump nicknamed "blue mass." Doctors tore off a chunk and gave it to the patient. Calomel also came in pre-measured doses in the form of pills called "blue pills."

The use of calomel produced feces that were a characteristic green color, and were thus called "calomel stools." The calomel stimulated the gall bladder to excrete copious amounts of bile into the intestines and thus turned the feces green.

Any form of mercury was irritating to human body tissues and, as one of the heavy metals, was highly toxic. Frequent doses of calomel could lead to chronic mercury poisoning. Undesired side effects of the "cure" included loss of memory, excessive salivation, various neurological problems, and disintegration of the teeth, gums, and bones. Overdose could also lead to shaking limbs, a condition that was called "mercuric trembling."

Earlier in the 1800s, mercury was used in the process of preparing beaver pelts for making hats. Those involved in the hat trade frequently developed the same strange neurological symptoms from breathing mercury fumes, hence the expression "mad as a hatter." Mercuric trembling was also found among workers who silvered mirrors with mercury.

Narcotic Drugs

Narcotic drugs were used to treat various ailments. Opium and morphine, which was derived from opium, were the primary drugs used for the relief of pain.

Opium

Opium had been used as a narcotic drug for hundreds of years and was a popular narcotic in the Old West in the nineteenth century. Opium, morphine, and cocaine were not controlled substances, as they are today. They were readily available over the counter in the Old West in local drugstores and were widely prescribed for a variety of ailments.[9] Opium and its medicinally-important derivative morphine, along with laudanum (a solution of opium in alcohol), were prescribed for pain control and for problems such as colds, fevers, consumption (tuberculosis), pleurisy, rheumatism, insomnia, cough suppression, and stomach disorders.

Opium and its derivatives were drugs of choice to treat dysentery and diarrhea because they relaxed the smooth muscles of the abdomen that propelled material through the intestinal tract. As one frontier physician succinctly put it, opium tended to "lock up the bowels."

Opium was made from the dried juice of the poppy plant *Papaver somniferum*, which was cultivated in China, India, and the near East. Opium arrived in China around A.D. 700 with Arab traders, where it was used as a pain medicine and to treat dysentery. Experimentation led to recreational uses. Smoking opium in China started in the 1600s to relieve boredom among the rich, and the drudgery of everyday life among the poor. As a result, the opium habit was commonplace in China in the 1800s.[10]

The recreational use of opium came to the United States with Chinese laborers who came to work in the California gold fields in the 1840s and 1850s, and later spread to those who worked on the construction of the western half of the transcontinental railroad between Sacramento and Omaha. From about

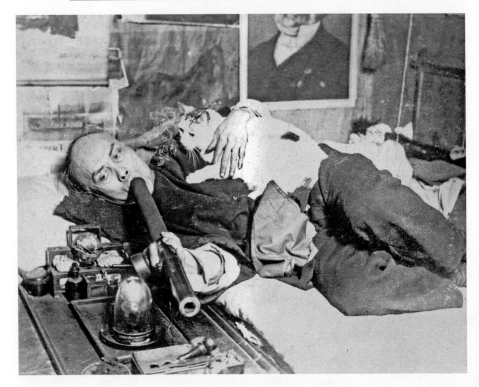

A Chinese man smoking an opium pipe, probably in California around 1890. His
collection of smoking paraphernalia is by his head (Denver Public Library Western History Collection, X-21494).

1850 to 1870 the practice of smoking opium remained primarily a Chinese
habit. During the 1870s, though, members of the underworld, such as pimps,
prostitutes, gamblers, and criminals, in California and Nevada started to use
it as a recreational drug.

The euphoria induced by opium slowly spread eastwards across the
country, and from the shady side of life, its use progressed to the suburban
housewife. Importation of opium increased steadily from 24,000 pounds in
1840 to 416,824 pounds in 1872.[11] Contemporary reports indicated that the
primary users of the drug were women. The trade grew and grew. In 1902 the
importation of opium increased to five times the amount imported in 1898.
In 1900, estimates were that 250,000 Americans were opium addicts. The
importation of opium from the Far East remained legal until 1906 and the
passage of the Pure Food and Drug Act. The Harrison Narcotic Act of 1914
ended the legal sale of narcotics over the counter.

The opium trade caused a ripple effect that even affected sea lions. Sea
lions off the coast of California were primarily hunted in the second half of

the nineteenth century for their blubber, which yielded valuable oil, and their skins, which were used for articles of clothing. Their unlikely association with the opium trade came when it was discovered that their whiskers were excellent for cleaning opium pipes. As if all this were not enough, males sea lions were also hunted for their testicles, which were dried and sold as aphrodisiacs.

As well as being used medicinally, opium continued to be smoked as a recreational drug. Opium dens were usually located in the Chinese section of a town, known as Chinatown, down a street often called "Hop Alley." These streets received the name because "hop" was a nickname for opium. Drug addicts were called "hoppies," and opium dens were called "hop joints." In the 1880s, Denver's Hop Alley, along Wazee Street, had twelve opium dens, with five more located on nearby streets. The mining town of Cripple Creek, Colorado, had a similar district.

Opium dens were all that Victorian literature would have readers believe. A series of tiny cubicles, furnished only with a cot to lie on, lined a dark, narrow corridor. The smoker or the den owner twisted a few drops of glue-like opium onto a wire loop and held it over an open flame. When the bead was sufficiently heated, it was rolled into a pill and placed in an opium pipe. The smoker lay on the cot, held the bowl of the pipe over an open flame, and inhaled the smoke from the heated opium. After a few puffs, the smoker passed into a hazy coma and faded into the pleasant dreams of the opium addict. A pill of opium typically cost between fifty and seventy-five cents.

Opium Derivatives

Opium contained over twenty-five alkaloids (derivatives of opium) that were used in medicine.[12] The most important was morphine, named after Morpheus, the Greek god of sleep. Morphine was first isolated from opium in 1803 by chemist Friedrich Sertürner in Germany. His initial publication went unnoticed until he published a second report in 1816.

Opium and morphine were widely used as painkillers on the battlefield during the Civil War, taken either as a pill or as powder applied directly to open wounds. An appropriate dosage was considered to be the amount of powdered morphine that would stick to a fingertip moistened by the doctor's saliva. To administer the dose, the powdered wet finger was pushed into the wound and the powder rubbed off.

Morphine was slow to be adopted as a painkiller because it was poorly absorbed in tissues and had limited effectiveness when administered by mouth. To offset this, however, a larger dose could be administered. For a greater tranquilizing effect, morphine was sometimes added to whiskey. It was not until the hypodermic syringe was invented and the drug could be injected directly into the bloodstream or under the skin that it became an important addition to the physician's roster of drugs.

Piston syringes for the injection of medication were available in the mid–1800s; however, the hypodermic needle had not yet been invented. Doctors had to make a small cut in the skin in order to be able to inject the medicine directly into the body. One of those to use this technique was Francis Rynd, who injected morphine dissolved in creosote as early as 1844. The first syringes had a point on the end, more in the form of a cone than a slender needle. The sharp end of the cone on these devices was pressed into the flesh, giving the nickname of the "painful point" to these early syringes.

In 1853, Charles Pravaz in France added a hollow needle to the end of an existing piston syringe to make a useful hypodermic device to inject substances under the skin. In 1855, Scottish physician Alexander Wood in Edinburgh used a fine, hollow needle, with a modified cutting point added, to inject morphine into the bloodstream to dull pain.

Before its addictive properties were understood, morphine was used as part of the treatment for alcoholism, and was even prescribed for hangovers. Doctors addicted alcoholics to morphine, thinking that morphine addiction was the lesser of the two evils. In similar fashion, morphine was used as part of the treatment for opium addicts. Morphine was also employed as a cough suppressant.

Heroin (diacetyl morphine — the so-called "heroic drug") was a highly addictive narcotic substance that was derived from morphine. First synthesized in 1898, it was commonly used for the treatment of asthma and coughs. Heroin was considered to be a non-addictive substitute for morphine and codeine, and heroin was used as a highly addictive cure for morphine addiction.[13]

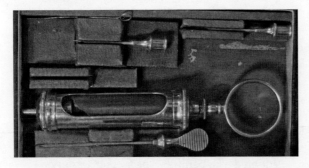

Early hypodermic syringes had to be cleaned after each use, but were a vast improvement for delivery of medication such as painkillers. The wire with the loop at the top was used for cleaning blood and matter out of the needles (author's collection).

Another important opium derivative was laudanum, which was a drinkable medicine made by dissolving opium in alcohol. Laudanum was commonly used as a sedative and painkiller. Also called tincture of opium, it was nicknamed "sleepy stuff," or "quietness." The use of this drug was not without its perils. As one contemporary medical manual warned, "The habitual use of tinctures and essences is full of danger. Many an invalid has unconsciously formed intemperate habits by means of these seductive medicines."[14]

Laudanum was used to treat headaches, toothaches, neuralgia (nerve pain), and was added to cough syrup. It was widely employed for "female complaints."

In large doses, laudanum and other narcotic drugs were used to commit suicide, particularly by disillusioned prostitutes. In 1883, twenty-one-year-old Sallie Talbot in Cheyenne, Wyoming, died a few hours after taking too much laudanum, in spite of the valiant efforts of Dr. W.A. Wyan. The same fate befell Laura Steele, a prostitute in Virginia City, Nevada, in 1875. A customer sleeping with Ida Vernon, one of the girls at Jenny Tyler's Bow Windows brothel in Virginia City, Nevada, woke in the morning to find that the thirty-two-year-old woman beside him was dead from an overdose of opium. Eleanor Dumont, known also as "Madame Moustache," gambled her way from Nevada City, California, to mining towns in Nevada and Montana, starting in the 1850s. Disillusioned by her waning fortunes, she swigged an overdose of morphine and was found lying by the roadside a few miles outside Bodie, California, on the morning of September 8, 1879.

Other stories had happier endings. Prostitutes Hattie Willis and Katie Thompson, who worked at Madam Rose Benjamin's bordello, tried to commit suicide using a combination of morphine and laudanum. Three doctors sprang to the rescue and pumped their stomachs. The women survived.

Paregoric, which was tincture of opium with camphor added, was used to treat asthma, to soothe teething babies, and to check diarrhea.

Cocaine

Cocaine (cocaine hydrochloride), derived from the leaves of the coca plant (*Erythroxylon coca*) that grew in Peru, was used as a local anesthetic to dull pain in the skin. It had little effect on unbroken skin, but was rapidly absorbed through the mucous membranes, such as the inside of the mouth, nose, and intestines, or through abraded or damaged skin, such as a wound. It was used primarily during minor surgical procedures as a local anesthetic for the nose, throat, or eye because it blocked nerve impulses and removed the sensation of pain. Lloyd's Cocaine Toothache Drops, for example, were used to relieve the pain of an aching tooth. Carl Koller of Vienna used cocaine in 1884 as a local anesthetic for eye operations, both to dull the pain and immobilize the eye muscles.

One of the oldest of the local anesthetics, cocaine was first isolated from coca leaves in 1859. It had many uses in the Old West, which also led to abuse. Before the full effects of the drug were known, early doctors and medical students performing experiments on themselves with cocaine often became addicted.

Cocaine was widely available, could be purchased over the counter in a drugstore, and appeared in many medicines. It was used in cough medicines, tonics, enemas, and poultices. It was used as a casual treatment for hay fever because the drug shrank inflamed tissues. To achieve the same effect, cocaine was used in the form of suppositories to treat rectal, uterine, and urethral diseases. One such medicine was Roger's Cocaine Pile Remedy, which was used to shrink the swollen tissues of painful hemorrhoids.

Whiskey

Whiskey was essentially ethyl alcohol (ethanol), with coloring and flavoring added during the distilling and aging process. While whiskey is no longer considered to be a drug, in the Old West it was looked upon as the universal drink and cure-all for almost any ailment or disease. Whiskey was referred to as grain alcohol because it was made from the fermented mash of various grains. It was also known medicinally by the grand name of *spiritus frumenti*. Medicinal brandy was known by the similar magnificent name of *spiritus vini gallici*.

Alcohol, in the form of fermented beverages, has been known since before recorded history. In the Old West it was thought to be the universal remedy. Drinking whiskey was considered by believers to strengthen the heart and lungs. Alcohol was also considered to be the cure for a wide variety of ailments, such as rabies, chills, heart palpitations, fever, and kidney disease. Among many others diseases, it was used for the treatment of dropsy, palsy, epilepsy, and jaundice. Sometimes whiskey was combined with quinine for the treatment or prevention of malaria. Emigrants on the Oregon Trail and soldiers at forts close to malaria breeding grounds took a daily dose of three grains of quinine in an ounce of whiskey as a preventative. Whiskey was also used as a painkiller, sedative, antiseptic, and disinfectant. Mixed with castor oil, it made a popular shampoo.

One interesting theory held that because alcohol was used to preserve biological specimens, drinking whiskey should similarly preserve the tissues of a heavy drinker and thus lengthen his life. Many alcoholics in the Old West experimented with this self-fulfilling concept — perhaps even if they didn't totally believe it.

Excessive alcohol consumption was believed to be the leading cause of spontaneous human combustion, which was one of the odder forms of injury and death reported by the Victorian press. Never explained satisfactorily, occasional reports surfaced in the newspapers of people spontaneously exploding with fire and being badly burned or even reduced to a pile of ashes. Clothing and nearby combustible objects were usually unscathed.[15]

As a more conventional remedy, alcohol was thought to be good for digestive problems. A drink of whiskey was considered good for the stomach to prepare for an upcoming meal, and was popular after the meal to help "settle" the digestion.

Some doctors prescribed whiskey to men with consumption to cheer their spirits and provide some relaxation from their gloomy ordeal. As a result, whiskey manufacturers promoted whiskey as a cure for tuberculosis— purely for medicinal use, of course. Many "lungers" became alcoholics after reading glowing advertisements in the local paper that promoted whiskey as a positive cure.

The general consumption of whiskey and other forms of alcohol was a common pastime for miners, loggers, cowboys, railroad construction workers, and other men who worked hard and played hard in the Old West. Drinking to the point of drunkenness was an accepted practice for men. Victorian women who appeared intoxicated in public were considered to be immoral, and heavy drinking by women was not a practice accepted by contemporary society. Many women, however, kept a bottle of whiskey among the kitchen supplies and could take a small drink or two if they felt the need (particularly for pain relief at "that time of the month"). If a woman did not drink,

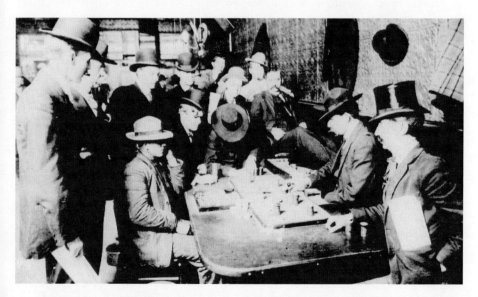

Drinking by men was an accepted practice in the Old West, as this convivial gathering around the gambling table at the Orient Saloon in Bisbee, Arizona, demonstrates (National Archives).

she might take an occasional swig of one of the many patent medicines that were available, most of which contained a high percentage of alcohol, and many of which were laced with opium or cocaine. Alcoholism in women was frowned upon, but taking a patent medicine or laudanum under a doctor's prescription was considered acceptable.

The incidence of alcoholism among men in the Old West was high. Heavy drinkers might put away a quart of whiskey a day. Bulbous red noses and eyeballs bloodshot with broken blood vessels were a common sight, and so was the shaking and tremors of *delirium tremens*. Not visible was the internal damage of cirrhosis of the liver, kidney damage, and the dulling of mental capacity. The severe form of alcoholism led to hallucinations and delusions, such as the feeling of snakes and spiders crawling all over the body.

Alcoholism was often a problem for women, though it was not as common as for men. Records from the Nevada State Hospital during the early mining era showed that a large number of women were institutionalized there for alcoholism and drug addiction.

More common than the use of alcohol for women was the use of opium. As well as being consumed by prostitutes and criminal women, it was the drug of choice for many middle-class women — some as young as fourteen. A quick swig from a bottle of laudanum could calm the nerves and settle the disposition. Estimates are that 60 to 70 percent of women of child-bearing age used opium, morphine, or laudanum for relief from menstrual or menopausal symptoms. Regular and sustained use of opium disrupted menstruation, and it is possible that this may have reduced the birth rate among prostitutes and other heavy users of opiates.

Whiskey was considered by residents of saloons and other drinking places to be a stimulant because it lowered inhibitions and gave the drinker a sense of euphoria. Excessive use of whiskey was equated by moral reformers with idleness, lying, and fraud. It was correctly associated by both groups with quarreling, fighting, obscenity, and moral problems.

In reality, alcohol was a depressant of the nervous system. It lowered mental capability and, in large enough quantities, acted as an anesthetic, producing unconsciousness. In moderate quantities, whiskey lowered many drinkers' sense of good judgment, concentration, and insight. At the same time, it made them excitable, impulsive, and argumentative. As a result, excessive use of alcohol was the basis for many gunfights in the Old West.

Often the participants of a gunfight were so drunk that they did not know what they were doing. As one example, when "Rowdy Joe" Lowe went after rival saloon owner "Red" Beard in Delano, Kansas, on the night of October 27, 1873, he was so drunk that he was not even sure that he had shot Beard. He had, because Beard died two weeks later from his wounds. Similar drinking to excess occurred when Warren Earp, Wyatt Earp's youngest brother, challenged Johnny Boyet to a gunfight after a dispute over a woman on July 6, 1900, in a saloon in Willcox, Arizona. Earp was so drunk that he forgot that he did not have his gun with him. Boyet aimed calmly and shot Earp in the chest.

During the Indian Wars on the Western frontier, the army had a particularly difficult problem with alcohol. Drunken soldiers were regularly involved in fights in saloons after payday, and visits to the post surgeon increased dramatically. Hangovers were also common the day after payday, and the guard house was full of hung-over miscreants. Castor oil was sometimes administered in large doses to men with hangovers to keep them up and about, so to speak.

It was not uncommon for enlisted army men and officers to be drunk on duty. An officer found drunk on duty might face a court martial, a suspension of rank or, if it was a serious or persistent problem, being cashiered from the service.

An enlisted man might receive fines or punishment that ranged from a reduction in rank to physical punishment, depending on the severity of the offense. He might also desert to stay one step ahead of retribution. Albert Barnitz, an officer in the Seventh Cavalry under General Custer, wrote in his journal on March 24, 1868, "My 1st Sergeant Francis S. Gordon was reduced to the ranks for absence without leave, and drunkenness, on the e'vg of 22d of March, and confined in the guard house." The next day, however, Barnitz wrote, "Serg't Gordon was released from the Guard House this morning, and at once absconded."[16]

Libbie Custer, General

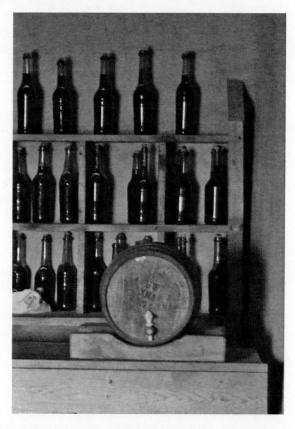

Homemade whiskey might show up in unlabeled bottles or in the keg in which the brew was made in the back room (author's collection).

Custer's wife, recalled one newly-transferred officer who came to visit her (as military protocol dictated regarding the commanding officer's wife). He had apparently celebrated a bit too much before observing his duties. When he arrived at her house, the man fell, rather than walked, through the door. After he stood up again, he proceeded to tangle his legs in his sword and fall over a chair. After an investigation, this impromptu alcoholic performance and breach of protocol caused him to resign his commission.

Attempts were made by the army to curb liquor and drunkenness among soldiers, but in most cases they were either unsuccessful or unenforced. In the 1880s, approximately 4 percent of army soldiers were hospitalized for alcoholism. Though this may not seem like a very large percentage, it occurred at a time when heavy drinking in the army was an accepted practice and alcoholism had to be extremely advanced for treatment to even be considered.

Alcoholism became such a problem for the army that the sale of whiskey on military reservations was banned in March 1881. This action, however, did not reduce the level of drinking as anticipated, but merely moved it off the post to nearby establishments, such as local saloons and hog ranches, which mushroomed just outside military limits and provided whiskey, gambling, and low-class prostitutes.

Whiskey in the Old West was not always the legitimate product, but could be easily manufactured in the back room of a saloon. Bootleg whiskey was made by starting with a fifty-gallon keg of ethyl alcohol, then adding various chemicals and flavorants until the result could fool inexperienced drinkers at the bar. Tobacco, tea, strychnine, soap, red pepper, prune juice, gunpowder, tree bark, and creosote were some of the additives used to give raw alcohol the general appearance of whiskey, along with an appropriate kick.

Drug Addiction

Opium, morphine, and cocaine were highly-addictive substances. Drug addiction was understood by 1880, but did not receive much attention until the 1890s. So many of the veterans that went home after the Civil War had been treated with opium for various ailments that opium addiction became known as the "old soldier's disease."

Though there were concerns about the problems of opium and morphine addiction, the damaging effects of the drugs were not fully understood, and treatments for various types of addiction used opium, morphine, and codeine as "cures."[17] For example, alcohol addiction and *delirium tremens* was often treated by the use of opium, and, perversely, morphine addiction was treated by the use of alcohol.

Some prostitutes routinely took a dose of laudanum or morphine every day so that they could cope with the grind of constantly entertaining men. This practice, of course, led to eventual addiction. Cases of addiction could be arrived at deliberately, but unknowingly, because some soft drinks and cigarettes were made with cocaine and morphine added in order to increase repeat sales of the product.

Drug overdoses, both intentional and accidental, were treated by pumping out the stomach before the drug had fully taken effect. An emergency first-aid remedy might be to make a semi-conscious victim swallow olive oil to coat the stomach and slow absorption of the drug, or mustard to induce vomiting. Among the more bizarre methods of treatment were injections of milk, severe flagellation, and attempted stimulation of a semi-conscious victim by the application of red hot irons to the feet.

If the time between the overdose and the treatment was delayed, and too much of the drug had been absorbed, nothing much could be done. One such unfortunate was Pearl De Vere, madam of the Old Homestead parlor house in Cripple Creek, Colorado. Whether she took morphine before going to bed to calm her nerves and took an accidental overdose, or whether she intentionally tried to commit suicide was never satisfactorily determined. What-

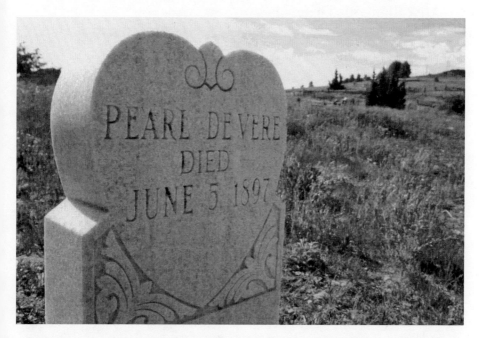

Here's how many purveyors of vice ended up. Madam Pearl De Vere of Cripple Creek, Colorado, died of an overdose of morphine, either intentionally or otherwise, on June 5, 1897 (author's collection).

ever the cause, Pearl was found on the morning of June 5, 1897, breathing heavily but unconscious. A local physician, Dr. Hereford, was summoned immediately, but the drug had been at work too long. He was unable to revive her, and she died several hours later.

Cocaine was another narcotic drug with the potential for abuse. Frequent recreational or medicinal use led to cocaine addiction. Unlike opium and morphine, cocaine was not physically addictive, but it produced a high level of psychological dependence. A moderate dose of the drug created the feeling of stimulation, well-being, and great mental power. Respiration rate and pulse were raised, and brain activity was increased. However, these sensations faded away rapidly and were followed by a feeling of deep depression. The solution for the addict was to ingest more cocaine and thus start a vicious cycle of mood swings between ecstasy and depression.

Cocaine overdose led to dizziness, fainting, and convulsions. Continued long-term use led to tremors, delirium, and insanity. A lesser problem for those who had reached this stage of addiction was gangrene of the inside of the nose.

Miscellaneous Drugs

One of the few effective early drugs was aspirin (acetylsalicylic acid), which was used to relieve pain. Salicylic acid was first developed in 1853 in Germany as a result of attempts to find a cheaper source of quinine than the *chinchona* tree. Though effective, this drug had some unpleasant side effects, and a similar drug, acetylsalicylic acid (or aspirin), was developed in 1895. It was not mass-produced, however, until the late 1890s by Bayer in Germany, making its use in the Old West limited. Cocaine was utilized instead to treat headaches and other aches and pains.

Another effective drug was ergot, derived from a parasitic fungus that grew on many species of moldy grain, particularly on rye, when the weather was warm and wet.[18] Ergot was chemically related to LSD (lysergic acid diethylamide) or "acid," a hallucinogenic drug that was prevalent for recreational use in the 1960s and 1970s. Ergot was used by midwives long before it became a drug recognized by doctors because it produced powerful contractions of the uterus. Ergot was administered in mild doses to stimulate childbirth and reduce bleeding afterwards. Large doses of ergot were utilized to produce miscarriages as a method of birth control, but its use for this purpose was often accompanied by serious toxic side effects. The plant filaree (storksbill, from the geranium family) and dried mistletoe were also employed by midwives to control excess bleeding after childbirth.

Strychnine, a poisonous material derived from the *Nux vomica* plant, was used medicinally as a tonic, a diuretic, and a laxative. In small doses it was utilized to stimulate the heart and the breathing. The dosage had to be regulated carefully, however, because overdoses of the drug caused muscle spasms that stopped the breathing and led to death. The use of strychnine was eventually discontinued as better drugs were found to replace all of its medical uses.

Counterirritants were substances that irritated the skin. A range of irritation was generated that ranged from those substances that merely reddened the skin to those that caused blistering and destroyed the skin tissue. A popular method of blistering was to apply a plaster of Spanish Fly (cantharides). A paste of this material was applied to the skin, then covered with a linen or leather wrap to produce large blisters over the desired area of treatment. Another method was to use poultices, which would apply moist heat to the body. Poultices were typically made with a burning-hot (often literally) ground flaxseed paste, perhaps mixed with wheat bran, applied to the skin. Flaxseed poultices could be made even more irritating to the skin by adding mustard flour. Boiling-hot water was sometimes poured over the affected part of the patient to achieve the same purpose.

While staying at Fort Laramie, Wyoming, Francis Parkman described how one of his companions treated an old Sioux woman for a case of eye inflammation brought about by too much exposure to the brilliant sun on the prairie. "A hideous, emaciated old woman sat in the darkest corner of the lodge, rocking to and fro with pain, and hiding her eyes from the light by pressing the palms of both hands against her face." Parkman described the doctor's reaction and makeshift blistering treatment:

> "It is strange," he said ... "that I forgot to bring any Spanish flies with me; we must have something here to answer for a counter irritant." So, in the absence of better, he seized upon a red-hot brand from the fire, and clapped it against the temple of the old squaw, who set up an unearthly howl, at which the rest of the family broke into a laugh.[19]

Tobacco was used as a medicine, primarily for the effects of the drug nicotine that tobacco contains. Tobacco was made from the dried leaf of a series of plants in the *Nicotiana* genus. Though primarily used for smoking or chewing, tobacco was also utilized as an insecticide (nicotine sulfate) and rat poison. Nicotine was so poisonous that tobacco was also used as an ingredient in sheep dip to kill parasites on the skin.

Folk medicine advised that a stream of tobacco juice or a wad of chewed tobacco placed on a cut would purify it. One of tobacco's primary medicinal uses came as a solution administered as an enema to treat intestinal worms. Tobacco was also used in cases of intestinal obstruction and strangulated hernias, where a loop of the intestine was obstructed and the blood supply cut off. Ingestion of large doses of nicotine caused tremors and convulsions, and, if large enough, caused death from respiratory arrest.

Nicotine was easily absorbed from the intestinal tract and, in small doses, had a stimulating effect on the nervous system, particularly on the respiratory system. As a result, one of the more curious uses for tobacco as a medicine was as a tobacco-smoke enema for the resuscitation of those who had apparently drowned. The smoke was applied via a device named a "fumigator."[20] Burning tobacco was placed in a metal box that had a rubber tube attached to each side of it. One tube ended in a nozzle that was inserted into the rectum; the other was attached to a pair of bellows that was used to blow the smoke into the patient. The technique was also used to revive lethargic newborn infants, women who had fainted, and to treat cases of asphyxiation.[21]

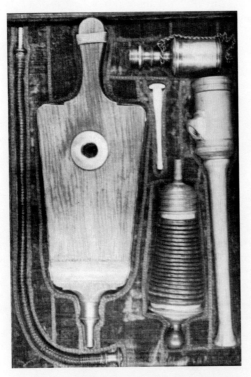

The vulgar old expression of "blowing smoke" took on new meaning when using one of these devices to resuscitate those who were nearly dead from drowning. The metal canister in the upper right was for burning the tobacco and was attached to the large bellows used to blow in the smoke (author's collection).

Colchicine, derived from the seeds and root of the plant *Colchicum autumnale* (meadow saffron) had been used for hundreds of years in the treatment of gout, a disease that caused pain and tenderness in the joints due to the deposition of uric acid. Gout was a common disease among the wealthy in the Victorian era, thought to be induced by excesses in eating and drinking habits.

Belladonna, derived from the deadly nightshade plant (*Atropa belladonna*), was another drug that had a long history, extending back to before Roman times. The name belladonna means "beautiful lady" and came from the practice of Roman women putting an extract of belladonna into their eyes to make them appear more beautiful. This practice was continued by prostitutes in the Old West because it dilated the pupils, made the eyes shine, and produced a healthy-looking flush in the cheeks. One undesirable side effect for the user was that the drug made it difficult to focus on objects close to the eye. In larger doses, belladonna was a stimulant, causing the user to become restless and talkative, also perhaps desirable attributes for ladies of the night. Belladonna was sometimes used to relieve symptoms of painful menstruation; however, only a fine line divided a safe dosage from one that produced collapse into a coma.

The drug digitalis was extracted from the dried leaves of the foxglove plant (*Digitalis purpurae*). It was used as a heart stimulant and a diuretic to remove water from the body in cases of dropsy, where fluid accumulated due to congestive heart failure. Digitalis worked as a diuretic not because it directly affected the kidneys, but because it improved heart action and, consequently, the circulation.

Drinking spring water that was heavily laden with sulfur and other minerals, from one of the fashionable spas, was considered to be the cure for everything from kidney and liver disorders to alcoholism. The drinker had to be determined because the water often smelled and tasted strongly of hydrogen sulfide — the same smell as rotten eggs. Water bottled from the Navajo Spring in Manitou Springs, Colorado, was so impregnated with the gas that workers had to wear safety masks when cleaning the water storage tanks at the factory. Their "Original Manitou Water" was bottled and shipped throughout the United States.

Chloral hydrate, first synthesized in the 1860s, was a mild sedative used as a potion to induce a period of sleep that resembled natural sleep. The drug acted fast, within ten or fifteen minutes, and produced a period of sleep that lasted five hours or more. It was an ideal drug for men with crooked intentions because it could be readily dissolved in whiskey, where it produced an additive effect to the depressant effect of the alcohol. Chloral hydrate was therefore known as "knock-out drops," "K.O. drops," or a "Mickey Finn" (hence the expression "to slip someone a Mickey"). After a shot or two of doctored whiskey in a crooked saloon or dance hall in a mining town, the drinker woke up sleeping on the ground in an alley with his pockets picked clean of gold dust.

In a similar manner, a man named Shanghai Kelly in San Francisco loaded up cigars with opium and gave them to visiting sailors who frequented his saloon. These loaded cigars were known as "Shanghai smokes." When a sailor had smoked enough to pass out, he was hauled out to a ship in San Francisco Bay (he was "shanghaied") and became part of a forced crew sailing for the Orient. Opium added to a drink of whiskey served the same purpose. Selling unwilling sailors to departing ships that were short of crew members was a flourishing business in major sea ports all up and down the Pacific Coast in the late 1800s.

CHAPTER SEVEN

Folk Remedies

By whatever manner it was achieved and maintained, one of the most valued possessions of the pioneers was good health, because daily life in the West involved hard physical labor in order to survive and succeed. Both men and women on a ranch or farm needed their health and strength. Routine daily chores, such as chopping wood, digging in the ground, and taking care of cows and horses, along with lifting and carrying heavy objects, such as saddles and hay bales, required a great deal of physical effort.

Men, in particular, needed strength and stamina to go about their daily work routine. Miners had to be able to dig and muck out gold and load ore cars; cowboys had to be able to ride for hours and wrestle recalcitrant cows; and loggers had to be able to fell and saw wood. Illness or ill health meant that they could not perform these tasks. The severity of an illness, in fact, was often judged by the degree of inability to perform daily work. A minor illness, such as a cold or rheumatism, was often borne in silence while continuing to perform the everyday jobs that had to be done. Of course, in the instance of serious illness or injury, some form of professional medical care was required.

As well as being treated with drugs prescribed by the conventional medical establishment, the men and women of the Old West self-medicated themselves with a variety of medicines of a different kind. These were the folk remedies—"cures" and medical wisdom that had been passed down from mother to daughter, typically consisting of herbal concoctions, potions, and salves. There were two primary reasons for this practice. One was the necessity for some sort of medical treatment in the absence of a doctor close at hand. The other reason was the result of the perceived high cost of conventional medical care.

The first reason that led to a high incidence of self-treatment was the scarcity of doctors on the frontier. In an emergency, the closest help for a pioneer living on an isolated ranch or in a remote mining camp might be themselves, a neighbor, or a spouse or friend. The nearest doctor might be a day's

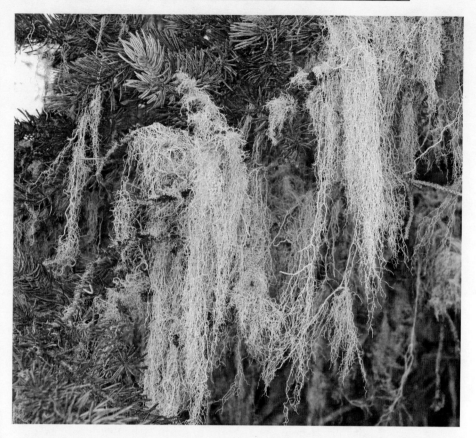

The thread-like qualities of Old Man's Beard, a lichen that grows on pine trees, was used as a folk remedy for packing a deep wound to stop severe bleeding. The plant also contained antibiotic properties, making it useful for suppressing the growth of bacteria at the same time (author's collection).

ride or more away. Out of necessity, many emergencies, such as broken bones, bleeding, choking, or snakebite, had to be treated as quickly as possible. In this situation, families had to be able to take care of themselves, at least in the early stages of a medical problem, until help could be summoned.

Wives were typically the primary source of home medical care, relying on themselves, a book containing home medical remedies, or a neighbor for additional assistance. A layman's book of medical advice, such as *Domestic Medicine: or, Poor Man's Friend*, first published in 1830 by Dr. John Gunn, served as a valuable medical reference for many pioneer wives.[1] Gunn's advice was apparently particularly welcome. By 1885, Gunn's book, which explained in simple layman's terms how to treat minor medical conditions, had reached its 213th edition.

These books were ideal for remote conditions on the frontier. They typically described themselves as "simply a household friend, which the inexperienced may consult on common occasions, or sudden emergencies, when medical advice is either unnecessary, or cannot be obtained."[2]

The second reason for pursuing self-treatment, rather than being tended by a professional doctor, was that a doctor's fees— modest though they might be — were often beyond the resources of a cash-strapped family. Many ranchers or farmers only had cash on hand at the end of the summer when they took their year's supply of beef or produce to market. In both of these instances, domestic manuals often served to provide medical advice. The doctor was sent for only as a last resort.

Another source of home medical advice were folk remedies that had originated within a family and been handed down from mother to daughter over several generations. These cures were often recorded in the family Bible or in mother's personal cookbook. In line with their cookbook origins, they were often called "recipes" or "receipts," both of which were early terms for what is now called a prescription. No matter how outlandish, a "cure" that appeared to work in a particular case of illness was often written down and then tried again when a similar case arose.

What these pioneer medical providers did not realize was that many diseases were self-limiting. That is to say, the patient's natural bodily defenses would spontaneously cure the disease after a few days, whether treatment was applied or not. Therefore, many bizarre treatments appeared to work and were regarded as effecting a cure. They were then recorded in the family medical guide or cookbook. Many of these recipes came from several previous generations of folk wisdom. As a result, unfortunately, the directions and opinions were not always up-to-date with current medical thinking.

In all fairness, some of the treatments applied did, of course, have a basis in healing abilities. Hot drinks, for example, did relieve congestion. Alcohol produced a feeling of soothing and relaxation. Baking soda was often useful in relieving a rash. Many of these pioneer remedies must have been effective. One doctor, William Allen, traveled west in 1851, hoping to set up a practice in Oregon City. But he found that there was little sickness among the hardy Oregon emigrants and not much demand for his services. To make ends meet he was forced to play his violin at local barn dances.

Chronic Conditions

Folk medicines were popular for treating minor chronic conditions. Aches and pains, colds and sniffles, and upset stomachs were constant companions of many of the pioneers, particularly those living in the cold, wet, harsh conditions of the mountains while they searched for their elusive pot of gold. Common complaints on the plains and in the mountains in wintertime were sore throats and runny noses due to frequently-occurring severe weather.

As men aged, prostate and kidney troubles became commoner. Because corrective surgical methods had not been developed, folk-inspired herbal medicines were frequently used in an attempt to promote an easier or more frequent flow of urine. As with most conditions, there were varied recommended folk methods of treatment. Among them, drinking the juice of artichokes mixed with white wine, eating cucumber seeds, eating the jelly from the inside of an unripe coconut, making a tea from the bark of the gooseberry bush, chewing asparagus roots soaked in water or mullein leaves steeped in water with strawberries, and eating pulverized juniper berries were all recommended cures. The list went on and on.

Arthritic conditions, such as rheumatism, which was often an affliction of older individuals who had worked at heavy physical labor for many years, were common. Typical cures for these aches and pains were concocted from the bark of the wild cherry tree, from angelica root, from horsemint herbs, coffee made from green berries, or tea made from the dried leaves of the sweet fern. A medicine that was presumably popular with many of the men (for a different reason) was a daily dose of two tablespoons of dandelion root and burdock root dissolved in gin. A similar treatment was to take the bark of a crabapple tree and dissolve it in "good" whiskey. The recommendation was to drink three wineglasses of this "medicine" each day until a gallon had been drunk or until good results had been obtained. Depending on the alcoholic taste of the patient, in some cases a "cure" probably took a while. One of the less-likely cures for rheumatism was the recommendation to throw a bean over the left shoulder into a well.

Skin conditions, such as warts and skin rashes, were common. Warts could supposedly be removed by washing the affected skin with a strong solution of washing soda. Alternate cures involved using a mixture of vinegar and baking soda, blistering the wart with Spanish Fly, wetting it with a solution of oak bark, or applying a paste of ashes and vinegar. One of the more drastic cures, which presumably worked by dissolving the wart, the underlying skin, and everything else in the area, was to daub the wart with a little oil of vitriol (almost pure sulfuric acid). One recommendation was to rub the wart with a slice of raw potato. A less conventional use for potatoes was to carry one in the pocket to cure rheumatism.

Bites were common in the outdoors and ranged from insect bites to tarantula and snake bites. Kerosene was recommended for bee stings. Vinegar or ammonia was used on spider bites. Snakebites, particularly on the Great Plains and in the sandy deserts of the Southwest, were common. Treatments were myriad. One popular notion was the application of warm manure to a snakebite. Perhaps more effective was to brew a tea from the prairie coneflower and pour it over the bite area.

The application of manure as a cure for different conditions was a common folk treatment. And not only cow manure was used. One recommendation for treating swelling was to rub the affected part with an ointment made by simmering chicken manure with onions in hog's lard.

A Cornucopia of Materials

Most of the home remedies consisted of the leaves, berries, roots, and flowers of various plants, and the bark of certain trees steeped in water or alcohol to make a liquid medicine, made into teas to be drunk hot, or made into a poultice or paste for direct application to the skin.[3] Mustard poultices and plasters were popular, and were applied to the chest to relieve coughs and croup, and wrapped around the limbs to relieve aches and pain.

Most remedies were taken by mouth or rubbed onto the afflicted part as an ointment. Some were administered as an enema. The reason for this alternate route of administration was that some remedies were not effective if given by mouth. Alumroot, for example (named after the astringent chemical alum used in pickling), was useful for treating cases of severe dysentery; however, if taken by mouth, its healing properties were neutralized during its passage through the small intestine. Therefore it had to be administered at the other end of the system, where it shrank inflamed tissues.

Many of these primitive plant extracts were the forerunners of the patent medicines that flourished during the last part of the nineteenth century. Part of the popularity for these medicines that eventually replaced home cures was that they were supposedly made from the same roots and natural herbs as the folk medicines that mother and grandma used.

Many household remedies relied on materials that were conveniently found around the farm or ranch. Therefore, materials such as lard, kerosene, mustard, vinegar, chicken fat, and whiskey were commonly used to compound folk medicines. Grease and oil, also common substances around a ranch, were utilized in many ways, from rubbing goose grease on the chest for colds to mutton tallow applied on rashes or rubbed on painful leg muscles for aches and cramps.

Oils and greases were particularly prized. Various animal oils were reputed to be particularly effective, and bear oil and grease were used in many preparations. One particularly aromatic oil was derived from skunks. One recommended use for this oil was that it be rubbed on the chest and throat in case of a chest cold. Liniment made from snake oil was reputed to be a

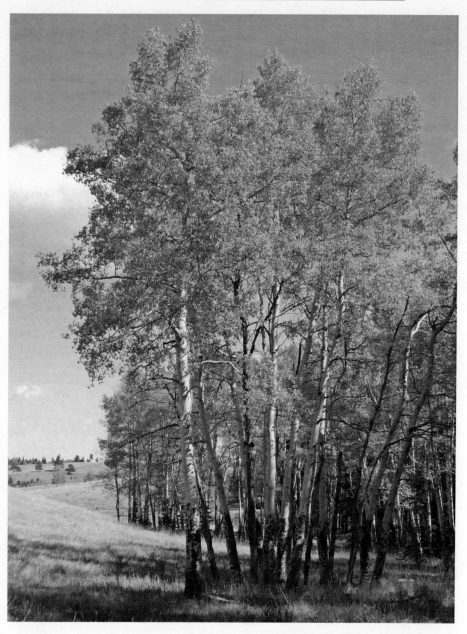

The bark of the aspen tree, which grew commonly in the Mountain West, contained a substance similar to aspirin, which could be extracted to relieve minor aches and pains. The white powdery substance covering the bark was used for a sunscreen. Another use for the bark was to soak it in sarsaparilla, then mix the resulting extract with whiskey. This drink was said to make a bracing tonic (author's collection).

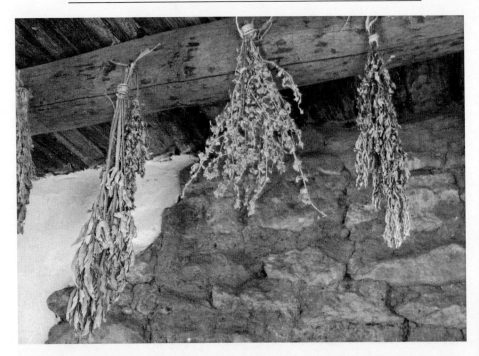

Medicinal herbs were gathered and then dried by hanging them from a nail in the rafters near the chimney, as in this adobe house in New Mexico. The dried plants were ground up for use (perhaps mixed with a little alcohol) (author's collection).

cure for rheumatism, sprains, and aching joints. It was also recommended as a sure cure for toothache.

Mountain men commonly used bear grease because it was available and handy in their way of life. It was employed for a variety of purposes, such as waterproofing clothes, as a salve for cuts and wounds, and by mouth as a laxative.

Vinegar found many uses, such as a gargle, a cooling drink when diluted with water, a treatment for nose bleeds, and a soothing wash for burns, rashes, and itches. Vinegar sprayed on the walls of a room was thought to ward off communicable diseases by acting as a disinfectant. It was also spread around liberally in a sickroom to cover up any unpleasant odors. One suggested cure for insanity was to rub vinegar on the head.

Another recommendation involving vinegar was to give a wineglassful of strong vinegar as a tonic to revive someone who was seriously drunk. It was said that this particular cure was often used by soldiers who had imbibed too much. Another folk remedy that was supposedly quite effective in reviving someone who was "helplessly intoxicated" was to have them drink a half-teaspoon of ammonium chloride in a glass of water. This remedy would allegedly "almost immediately restore the faculties and powers of locomotion."[4] One would think so.

Tobacco, being a common item around the ranch or farm, was frequently used as an ingredient in various folk medicines. It was smoked with the dried leaves of the jimson weed (Jamestown weed or datura, one of the nightshade family) for relief of difficult breathing. Perverse as this treatment sounds, it actually had some merit. The combination acted to relieve bronchial spasms by temporarily numbing the bronchial nerves and drying up excess fluid in the membranes of the lung. Jimson weed was also combined with mullein leaves and smoked for the same purpose.

Combined with vinegar and lye, tobacco was used as a wash for ringworm, which is a painful itchy skin condition caused by a fungus. One variation on this treatment was to boil tobacco in urine, then mix it with lye and vinegar. This mixture was to be frequently applied to areas affected with ringworm. In this case, the application of tobacco may have been beneficial, as the nicotine contained in tobacco was a poisonous material. Tobacco was combined with fresh butter to make a poultice to be applied to hemorrhoids. Another hemorrhoidal treatment using tobacco consisted of a mixture of tobacco juice, sulfur, and hog's lard combined into an ointment. Tobacco was administered as an enema for relief from bilious complaints. Combined with spikenard root and comfrey root, it was boiled with lye and made into a salve for sore breasts.

Some conditions brought out a host of cures. The treatment of asthma, for example. Among some of the recommended cures were sniffing borax up the nose, eating a spoonful of molasses mixed with crushed roasted eggshells three times a day, stuffing the sufferer's pillow with dried elder leaves, rubbing goose oil on the chest, drinking white daisy blossoms steeped in boiling water, or drinking an ounce of bloodroot dissolved in gin. One pioneer folk remedy consisted of simmering skunkcabbage root in hen's fat and then taking a teaspoon of the mixture three times a day. Perhaps a more palatable mixture was skunkcabbage root and rock candy steeped in boiling water, then mixed with an equal quantity of whiskey and drunk by the shot-glassful. A few of the asthma cures would seem to have no discernible merit, such as the recommendation of wearing a muskrat pelt with the fur side next to the skin in order to gain relief.

One simple treatment for dandruff was to massage the scalp with coal oil.[5]

Other Treatments

There was very little home surgery, but treatment could involve setting broken bones, cutting off calluses, or sewing up bad cuts and tears in the flesh.

If injuries did occur, they often had to be treated in a timely manner in order to prevent serious bleeding or the onset of gangrene. When a man named Andrew Broadus accidentally shot himself in the arm during a buffalo hunt out on the Plains in southwest Kansas, he was far from any professional medical help. In his case, infection set in after a few days and it was necessary to amputate the arm to save his life. His friends reluctantly agreed to help. One operated using a shaving razor to cut away the putrefied flesh, while another cut through the bone with a handsaw. A third cauterized bleeding blood vessels with an iron bolt that was heated in the coals of a fire, while the other two men cut. The stump of his arm was sealed with tar to stop the bleeding. In spite of this crude treatment, Broadus survived and recovered fully.

A holdover from Hippocratic medicine, the idea of "impure blood" was still common among the public during the mid-to-late 1800s. Home remedies to supposedly counteract this condition included drinking copious amounts of sassafras or other herbal teas in the spring and fall to "purify" the blood. From this deeply-rooted idea, it was only a small step for the purveyors of patent medicines to offer potions that offered to cleanse "impure blood." Sassafras, incidentally, must have been a multi-purpose tea. One manual of folk remedies suggested using it to thin the blood; another to thicken the blood.

As well as a need to cleanse the blood, another common idea was that the body required periodic cleansing, particularly in the spring after a long winter of living inside, away from nature's fresh air and healing sunshine. Impurities needed to be sweated out of the skin, the kidneys needed to be well-flushed, and the bowels needed to be purged. Mother's natural remedies provided for this obsession with the stomach and bowels. Powdered rhubarb, mixed with ipecac and soap, was said to make an excellent tonic for an upset stomach that "leaves the stomach braced." A tea made from the sage bush was said to be a good treatment for "weak and windy stomachs."

Many folk medicines were touted as emmenagogues, or drugs that stimulated menstrual flow. Among them were bloodroot, comfrey, and tansy (part of the aster family).

Folk cures were also applied to infectious diseases, even though the concept of viruses and bacteria as disease agents was not known. For example, several herbal cures were recommended for measles. One of the more peculiar treatments for the disease was to eat a roasted mouse. For some unstated reason it had to be cooked to a well-done state.

Nose bleeds could be stopped by the sensible procedure of plugging up the nostril with clean cotton. A more bizarre treatment was to insert a chunk of pork to stop the bleeding. Whether the pork was to be cooked or used raw was not specified.

Even then, the simple concept of a nosebleed resulting from a broken blood vessel was not properly understood. There was a great reluctance to discard the old theories of bleeding and purging as treatments. As late as 1852, one book of home remedies emphatically stated:

> The idea of this [nosebleed] proceeding from the ruptured blood vessels is ridiculous: it is a means taken by nature of thoroughly depleting a part so as to cure disease. It was no doubt in consequence of observing these sanguineous depletions of nature, that the idea originated of doing it artificially, and thence the introduction of blood-letting in all its various forms of abstraction.[6]

Bleeding was still recommended in some of the home manuals of the mid–1800s as a cure for fever. One home medical book said, "Bleeding from the arm ... to fainting, will often cut short the disease at once."[7]

The concept of purging was also held over from early Hippocratic medicine. One recommendation was a dose of ten grains of jalap combined with thirty grains of cream of tartar (potassium acid tartarate — a reddish sediment precipitated out during the fermentation of wine), which would seem to be a large dose.[8] The instructions noted that after taking this, "[The] bowels should be well purged."[9]

The ears and hearing were not immune from folk medicine. Deafness was treated by blending ant's eggs with onion juice and pouring the mixture into the affected ear. One reputed cure for earache was to take an onion and wrap it in tobacco leaves, then, after baking the combination, squeeze out the juice and pour it into the external ear canal. A cure for earache that sounds more reasonable was to wet cotton wool with olive oil and paregoric, and insert the cotton into the ear. One folk cure for ear infection was to mix the powdered leaves of the mullein plant with olive oil and pour it into the ear canal. Similar to the cure for nose bleeds, one recommendation for earache was to insert a wedge of salt pork (for this cure, lightly toasted) into the ear canal. A less appealing cure for earache was warm urine poured into the ear.

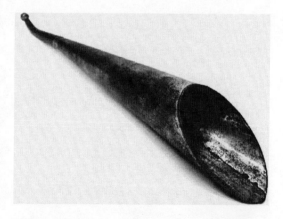

In spite of peculiar folk remedies, help for hearing problems was limited. One solution was to use an ear trumpet, such as this primitive tin device, to collect sound and funnel it into the ear (author's collection).

Human urine was used for a variety of other treatments. It was rubbed onto sore skin, poured into inflamed eyes, and daubed on the face to improve the complexion. Lameness was treated by combining a pint of urine, a table-spoon of salt, and a small amount of tobacco to make a wash for sore feet. The instructions speak for themselves: "in using the wash, if it should cause nausea, take one tea-spoonful of the tincture [of guaiacum] and cease bathing."[10]

Drowning, or near-drowning, was not an unusual occurrence because swimming was not the popular pastime that it is today, and the ability to swim was not universal. Interestingly, several home medical manuals from the mid-nineteenth century recommended an early method of mouth-to-mouth resuscitation, describing blocking the victim's nose and breathing into the victim's mouth to ventilate the lungs. However, if this method failed, the instructions went on to recommend an enema of turpentine, a very irritat-ing substance. If anything would wake the near-drowned, presumably that would. Other stimulating treatments for drowning called for snuff or ginger to be blown up the nose.

And finally, impotence was always one of the darkest fears of the Victo-rian male. Part of the reason that sarsaparilla was popular as a frontier drink may have been that folk medicine gave it the reputation for restoring sexual vigor and performance to aging men.

CHAPTER EIGHT

From Sawbones to Surgeon

Though doctors in the Old West may have had difficulty diagnosing and curing many of the infectious diseases that they encountered, they had reasonable success in treating physical injuries. The hazards of daily life in the Old West meant that many of the doctor's treatments were of a surgical nature, such as treating gunshot and arrow wounds, broken bones, and miscellaneous cuts and bruises. Some wounds were due to accidents, such as sharp tools and knives, mishaps with axes, falling off a horse, or being gored by a rampaging steer. Others were the result of attacks by hostile Indians or from another man's bullets.

The impact of soft lead bullets from gunshot wounds, in particular, created tremendous bodily damage, ripping flesh and producing shattered and splintered bones. Doctors would probe the bullet hole to discover the extent of the injuries, as well as to remove embedded fragments of lead bullets and clean out debris carried into the wound. In cases of serious wounds to the torso, very often all the doctor could do was try to stop any major bleeding and prescribe morphine for pain.

Most surgical procedures in the early days of the frontier were performed in the patient's home. Hospitals were lacking, and even when they became more widespread, patients often preferred to stay at home. Part of the difficulty was the transportation of sick or injured patients in outlying areas of the rural West to a hospital in town. In addition, there was no real need for a patient to go to a hospital. X-rays and today's sophisticated medical and laboratory tests were unknown. Diagnosis was provided in the home by the doctor's senses of sight, hearing, smell, and touch. Nursing care could be provided by the patient's family.

When hospitals became more widespread, gathering patients there was often initially more for the convenience of the doctor, who could treat all his patients at a common location instead of making his rounds to widely separated ranches or farms. As x-rays and laboratories came to play a large role in diagnosis, and antiseptic surgery became routine, it became more important for a patient to be admitted to a hospital to receive the best possible care.

Surgical Instruments

The doctor's operating kit included a fearsome-looking array of instruments. Amputation saws, curved and straight amputation knives, scissors, forceps, retractors, probes, artery clamps, scalpels, bone nippers, a leather tourniquet, and a large hacksaw figured prominently among the surgical tools. One gruesome-looking instrument was a tenaculum, a probe with a hooked point to snag and draw an artery out of the flesh for closing it off with a suture.

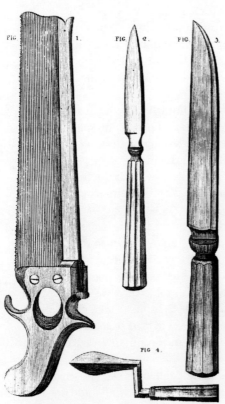

Early surgeons in the Old West operated while wearing their regular street clothes. Bloodstains and other marks on the clothing from operations were worn proudly as a badge of success for a good surgeon.

Surgical gowns, but without a mask or cap, came into use in the operating theater starting in the 1890s. The introduction of rubber gloves for surgery was originally not for sterility but to prevent hand irritation among operating room nurses. The mercuric chloride solution that doctors and nurses used for washing their hands before undertaking surgery was highly irritating to the skin. To try to overcome this problem, in 1890 William Halsted, a professor of surgery at Johns Hopkins Medical School, asked the Goodyear Rubber Company to make some thin rubber gloves to protect the nurses' hands. The initial gloves, which could be sterilized, were a great success, and Halsted soon outfitted his entire surgical team with them. Word of this success spread, and their use was quickly adopted by other surgeons.

Early surgical implements consisted primarily of instruments to perform amputation, such as this gruesome-looking bone saw and sharp amputation knives (National Library of Medicine).

Amputation

In the 1850s, surgical techniques were not suitable, or safe, for operations that penetrated major body cavities, such as the chest or abdomen. A ruptured appendix or a perforation of the bowel was generally not diagnosed until acute abdominal infection (peritonitis) had set in and it was too late for a cure. The generic cause of death in these cases was listed as "inflammation of the bowels." Such was the diagnosis of death for Alfred Packeral, a young English miner who died in Tombstone in 1882.

The commonest type of surgery was amputation for wounds of the extremities or to treat compound fractures, where fragments of bone protruded through the skin. A simple fracture of an arm or leg, where the broken ends of the bone did not pierce the skin, was usually treated with a splint to immobilize the bone until the ends knitted together. A compound fracture was far more serious because of the risk of infection through broken skin. A further danger for the patient was that transporting a patient with a simple fracture to medical care in a bouncing wagon or in an army ambulance with no springs could easily turn a simple fracture into a compound fracture.

As well as being a "cure" for compound fractures, amputation was used to treat uncontrollable bleeding in an arm or leg, severe laceration or crushing of soft tissue in the extremities, extensive damage to nerves or blood vessels, foreign material that was deeply embedded in a wound, or a bullet wound that involved one of the joints, such as a knee or elbow. Hertzler remembered a lacerated hand being treated by amputation.[1] Amputation was typically not used for gunshot injuries to hands, arms, or legs, if the underlying nerves and blood vessels had undergone relatively little damage.

Amputation, though a drastic measure, might be performed if the victim of an accident was located on a remote ranch or some other distant place where there was nobody present to care for the injured person. The thinking was that if amputation was not performed, the person would die from infection. In reality, the amputation procedure might itself induce an infection that would kill the patient anyway.

The smaller the body part to be amputated, the better the patient's chance of survival. Nearly all patients survived the amputation of a finger or a toe. The fatality rate for the amputation of an arm was about 20 percent. Operations that involved a joint, such as a shoulder or knee, had a higher fatality rate because joints were highly susceptible to infection during surgery. The worst survival rates were for amputation of the whole leg, particularly when performed at the thigh. More than three-quarters of those who underwent leg surgery died due to a massive loss of blood and the high risk of post-surgical infection.

Amputation was a crude procedure. Before anesthetics were developed for surgery, patients were conscious during the entire procedure. As a result, the most important skill of a surgeon was speed. Because of the agony involved for the patient, medical students and operating-room assistants were often selected for their brawn rather than their brains. But even then, they could only hold a patient steady for a few minutes during surgery. But that might be long enough. Fast surgeons could cut away tissue, saw a bone in two, and tie off bleeding blood vessels within the space of only two or three minutes.

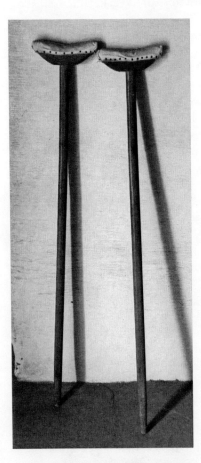

As well as amputations, broken legs and sprained ankles were common when dealing with livestock and operating heavy equipment. Victims had to hobble around on home-made crutches like these (author's collection).

The amputation procedure was started by strapping a tourniquet around the affected extremity above the planned area of surgery in order to compress the underlying artery and control bleeding. Then the surgeon performed a quick circular cut with a curved knife through the flesh and muscles surrounding the limb. He made either a straight cut down to where the bone would be sawn, or he retracted the flesh for one to two inches above the point where he would saw in order to create a flap of skin to later cover the end of the remaining bone. Next, an assistant retracted the cut flesh, and the surgeon quickly sawed through the bone. The practice of amputation was so common that it led to the generic nickname of "sawbones" for a doctor.

Amputation was typically performed within the first twenty-four to forty-eight hours following an injury. After that time, infection often set in during what was called the "irritative stage" because the fever or swelling of infection usually started from forty-eight to sixty hours after the wound was received. After about forty-eight hours, any attempts at surgery spread infected material into undamaged tissue, contrary to what was desired, thus lessening the patient's chances of survival.

Surgeons did not always operate immediately because they thought that a patient in shock from blood loss should be allowed to rally before they operated. If the surgery was delayed for some reason, the chances of recovery were diminished by the increased likelihood of infection and blood poisoning, so attempts were sometimes made to "rally" the patient faster by administering whiskey.

If an injury or bullet fractured a bone in an arm or leg, a deliberate decision was sometimes made not to amputate, and an attempt made to save the limb. This alternative to amputation was resection, which was also called "excision." This was a surgical procedure in which bone fragments were removed and the remaining wound in the flesh was sewn up and allowed to heal. Unfortunately for the patient, removing a shattered section of bone also removed support for the remaining limb. Without skeletal support, and with an accompanying loss of nerves and muscle, a healed arm often dangled uselessly by the patient's side.

Resection was not a popular procedure because it involved a more complicated operation than amputation, it took longer to perform, and it had a slightly higher rate of mortality. In most cases the limb had to be amputated later anyway. Considering these reasons, most surgeons preferred to amputate.

Infection

Until the 1880s, the most severe problem associated with surgery, and the one that most often led to death, was the risk of infection. Infection after an operation occurred almost inevitably, though the causes for it were not understood at the time. Doctors realized that the inflammation of wounds was somehow connected to a progression of illness that often led to gangrene and death, but they didn't understand that the inflammation was the result of bacteria. The presence of bacteria could be observed through a microscope (if one was available), but this was interpreted, along with an increase in white blood cells, as part of the healing process. Surgeons scraped away as much dead tissue as they could, but infectious material often remained anyway.

Infection was caused by *Staphylococcus* and *Streptococcus* bacteria that contaminated broken skin after surgery. The result was pus, which was composed of dead cells, bacteria, and decomposed tissue that oozed from an infected wound.

Staphylococcus infection — also called the "pus producer" — was a common source of surgical infection, but wounds with this type of infection healed acceptably in most cases. The occurrence of pus due to *Staphylococcus* infection was considered to be one of the signs of healing and was greeted with enthusiasm by surgeons as "laudable pus." Even after the causes of infection were identified, the presence of "laudable pus" was still considered to be a good sign on the road towards healing. Wounds that healed without pus were considered to be medical curiosities. The associated negative aspect was that the discharge of pus attracted house flies, which laid their eggs in wounds and filled them with maggots (the juvenile form of flies).

Streptococcus infection had a higher death rate than *Staphylococcus* infections due to blood poisoning. Erysipelas was a severe skin infection from *Streptococcus* bacteria that entered the body through a break in the skin, such as a cut or abrasion, and led to blood poisoning.

Infection contracted during surgery was called "surgical fever." Infection contracted after surgery was called "hospital gangrene" or "ward gangrene"—a virulent form of *Streptococcus* infection. Both were highly infectious.

The inflammation that accompanied infection was thought to be due to "nervous irritability," "over-excitement" in the body, or "nervous congestion" of the blood. One treatment for infection, therefore, was the old

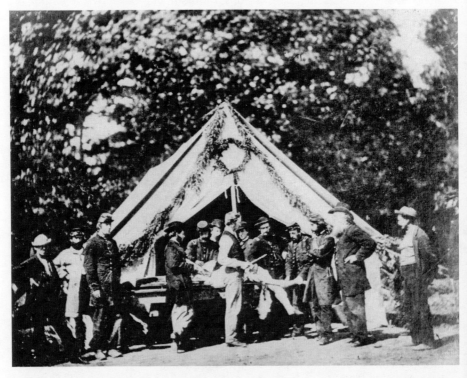

Amputation being performed in a tent at Gettysburg in 1863. The outdoor setting and curious onlookers surrounding the surgeon both contributed to a lack of sterility during the operation (National Archives).

standby—bleeding (along with purging, sweating, and vomiting) to remove "impurities." The greater the swelling, pain, and inflammation, the more the patient was bled to reduce the "over-excitement." Another treatment was the use of hot poultices to relieve pain, and reduce the swelling and discharge of pus.

In reality, in many cases the surgeon introduced infectious agents through non-sterile surgical methods. Infection was spread by unclean hands, by instruments and sponges that were not disinfected, and by unwashed dressings contaminated with pus from previous use. Surgeons often probed chest and abdominal wounds for a bullet or cleaned debris out of a wound with their bare unwashed fingers, spreading infection as they did so. Once infection set in and was diagnosed, surgeons attempted to cure it, but antiseptics, such as carbolic acid, might not be applied until after a wound had become infected, and by then it was often too late to save a patient dying from blood poisoning.

Surgical instruments were not routinely disinfected, even the metal probes used to locate bullets within a wound and the retractors used to open wounds for inspection and cleaning. Methods for disinfecting surgical instruments with bromine solution, carbolic acid, sodium hypochlorite (chlorine bleach), and bichloride of mercury were known at mid-century; however, this practice was not generally followed because most surgeons in the 1860s still thought that infection was caused by a noxious miasma in the air. Because this supposed infectious agent was already in the air, they felt that the surgeon had nothing to do with introducing infection to the patient. A few surgeons boiled surgical instruments to sterilize them, but the practice was not widespread.

Arthur Hertzler remembered this experience from his early days as a doctor: "In the first operation I witnessed the surgeon threaded the needles with silk and then stuck them in the lapel of his coat so as to have them readily accessible when needed. He held the knife in his teeth when not in actual use."[2] Some doctors moistened the end of surgical thread with their own saliva in order to be able to thread it easily into the eye of the needle before sewing up a wound.

The man who finally linked the presence of bacteria to infection was Ignatz Semmelweis, a physician at the General Hospital of Vienna. In the late 1840s he observed that there was a high rate of deaths in the obstetrical ward where women were attended by student doctors, as opposed to the ward where they were attended by midwives. He also noted that childbirth fever exhibited the same symptoms and progression as wound infection. After careful investigation, he linked the high rate of infection to doctors and medical students who performed dissections and autopsies, then continued on to examine obstetrical patients without washing their hands. Surgical dressings were usually reused and were not always washed after use, thus further spreading infection.

Semmelweis insisted that the wards be scrubbed clean, and that doctors and medical students wash their hands with a chlorine solution as a disinfectant to eliminate germs before examining patients. With these routine precautions in place, the death rate in the doctor's ward soon dropped from an average of 15 percent to around 1 percent. However, these findings were rejected by the hospital, and Semmelweis left his post in 1850. He moved to

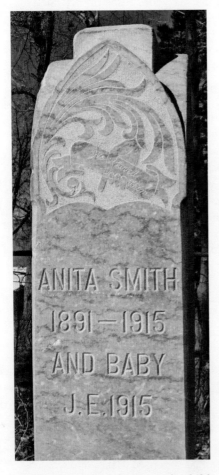

Deaths of mother and child (buried here in a common grave) during childbirth, or shortly after due to child-bed infection, were not uncommon (author's collection).

another hospital in Budapest to practice obstetrics and published his findings in 1855, but it was the 1870s before his theory of infection was widely accepted. Others, including renowned American physician Oliver Wendell Holmes, had theorized from similar findings before Semmelweis, but had not pursued it because of resistance to the concept. Semmelweis pursued and proved the concept in spite of keen opposition to his ideas.[3]

In spite of positive proof, however, some doctors were reluctant to accept the germ theory. Arthur Hertzler commented that when he was practicing, a high proportion of women in a particular vicinity died of childbirth fever. Primarily they were patients of a doctor who also raised pigs. As Hertzler described it, "[This doctor] sometimes washed his hands after the completion of labor but never before. After making a digital examination, he used his pants ... as a towel."[4]

Sterilization

The champion of the sterilization of wounds, surgical instruments, and hospital rooms was English surgeon Joseph Lister. In his medical practice, Lister noticed a difference in death rate in patients with simple fractures and those with compound fractures. Those whose skin had been pierced by broken bone contracted far more infections that were deadly. French chemist Louis Pasteur had recently shown that bacteria were present everywhere in the air, so Lister theorized that some of these germs entered a patient's body via the broken skin and caused infection. Lister tested his theory on August 12, 1865, while operating on an eleven-year-old boy, James Greenlees, whose leg had been fractured when he was run over by the wheel of a cart. Lister sprayed the wound, the operating instruments, the operating theater, and even the surgeon with carbolic acid as a disinfectant.[5] The technique worked, and Lister published his results on routine carbolic acid antisepsis for surgery in 1867. Lister's carbolic acid spray techniques did not receive widespread acceptance until the 1870s and were replaced in the 1880s by better methods of sterilization.

Eventually it became apparent that the infectious agents were not specifically in the air but were everywhere else on surfaces in the operating room. By 1890 Lister's carbolic acid spray was discontinued when it was found that cleanliness of the surgical instruments, the surgeon's clothing, the operating room, and bandages was more important. Thorough washing of hands and clothing was instituted as a critical part of the preparation for a surgical procedure.

Another positive outcome from Lister's work was a change in the design of surgical instruments. Scalpels and other similar surgical instruments were originally made with wooden handles. These instruments were subsequently redesigned to be totally metal so that they could be completely sterilized before use.

Other Surgery

At mid-century, and for several decades afterwards, surgical operations on the abdomen, chest, and brain were extremely risky and rarely performed. Abdominal wounds that penetrated the small intestine or stomach were almost invariably fatal. Wounds that entered the large intestine were fatal about 90 percent of the time. Those with chest wounds had a somewhat better chance of survival, but about 60 percent of the time died anyway.

The primary reason that such surgery was extremely dangerous was the threat of infection. Procedures that today are relatively simple, such as an appendectomy or operations to remove a gall bladder or ovarian cyst, almost inevitably resulted in death from peritonitis. In his autobiography, Arthur Hertzler recalled that his grandfather died of a strangulated hernia, where a loop of bowel is trapped and the blood supply cut off. This condition is easily repaired today. At that time it was considered inoperable. Hertzler made the chilling comment, "I can still hear his continued vomiting for the ten days he lived."[6]

Only a few surgeons explored the abdomen before the 1880s and 1890s. Even then, their basic procedure was simply to open the abdominal cavity, allow any infectious products to drain out, irrigate the inside to clean it out, and hope for the best. Even though this was a risky procedure, by the same token, not doing anything was also usually fatal. For example, appendicitis (then called "inflammation of the bowels") usually resulted in death if not treated. Before the appropriate surgery was developed, one treatment was the use of enemas or a large "dose of salts," such as Epsom salts, until the bowels moved. Modern medicine would not countenance this treatment, as it could cause the inflamed appendix to burst and cause deadly peritonitis. The first successful appendectomy was performed in 1883 in Davenport, Iowa, by Dr. W.W. Grant. This broke the barrier of abdominal operations, and surgeons went on to operate on gall bladders and hernias, and perform various gynecological procedures.

Infection could arise from any non-sterile, invasive procedure. For example, enlargement of the prostate in men was treated by the use of metal or rubber catheters forced into the urethra. At some point these continued treatments with non-sterile instruments resulted in kidney infection, which eventually killed the patient.

Another tricky surgical task was repairing injuries to the head. Depressed fractures of the skull were not uncommon due to accidents or from deliberate blows to the head during fights or military campaigns. Broken parts of the skull were treated by surgery that used a trephine, which was a cutting saw that drilled a circular hole in the skull. Early cutting blades had the shape of a cylinder; as a result, they often perforated the dura mater — the protec-

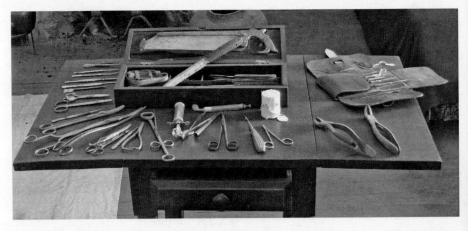

These instruments laid out on the operating table, ready for a surgical procedure in a doctor's office, illustrate the definite lack of sterile preparation and storage of instruments (author's collection).

tive covering of the brain — when the surgeon drilled through the bone. Later saw blades were shaped like a tapered cone to prevent the serrated blade from going too deep and damaging brain tissue when the saw broke through the skull. Other specialized tools were used to trim the ragged edges of the hole in the remaining bone after it was opened and to remove any bone fragments. Following surgery, the hole in the skull was typically covered with a metal plate, often made of silver or gold, that did not react with body tissues.

A good surgeon also had to know when not to operate. Observing the patient and not risking the infection and other complications that often followed surgery was sometimes a wiser course of action.

Anesthesia

Before the development of anesthesia, a major obstacle to successful surgery, whether it was for gunshot wounds, illness, or injuries, was the severe pain involved for the patient.[7] This drawback restricted the scope of surgery and made speed essential for the limited types of surgery that could be performed. Before the introduction of anesthesia, both doctor and patient viewed surgery as a last resort. It was typical for both to wait until an illness developed to the point where a life-or-death decision had to be made before the patient would agree to be cut open.

Early surgeons in the Old West doped up their patients with whiskey, opium, laudanum, or brandy to produce some nominal relaxation from nervousness and tension, and to at least partially dull the agony of the surgical procedure. If nothing else was available, a block of wood or leather was sometimes used for the patient to bite on, to try and help alleviate the suffering as they clenched their jaw at painful moments during the surgery. Under primitive conditions, a bullet might be used, hence the old expression of "biting the bullet." In spite of the heroic legends of the Wild West movies and novels, this method was actually uncommon, and the use of anesthesia was widespread both during the Civil War and on the Western frontier.

By the 1830s, doctors realized that some method of tranquilizing the patient would be beneficial to avoid or reduce protracted pain during surgical operations. Two likely candidates were nitrous oxide and ether. These chemical substances were already known to have the appropriate properties for dulling pain and were being used as recreational drugs by the public. Participants in what were called "frolics" soaked a cloth in ether and inhaled the vapors to induce a feeling of euphoria and well-being. Nitrous oxide was used in a similar manner at "laughing gas parties."[8] In the participants' intoxicated state, the side effects included staggering and odd behavior; but at least they apparently felt no pain if they injured themselves when they fell down or inadvertently ran into surrounding objects. In light of this, the anesthetic properties of ether and nitrous oxide were developed for use in the operating room.

Several doctors and dentists used nitrous oxide and ether for anesthesia in the early 1840s, and it is difficult to confirm with accuracy who was the first. William Clarke, a student at Berkshire Medical College, was one of the first in the United States to use ether in a dental procedure when he assisted Elijah Pope to extract a bad tooth from a patient in January 1842. The same year, physician Crawford Long of Jefferson, Georgia, also used ether for dulling pain in several minor surgical procedures. William Thomas Morton, a Boston dentist who later studied medicine, applied ether to a tooth he was going to drill and observed that the patient's entire mouth became numb. Morton was one of the first to successfully demonstrate the use of ether during surgery when he anesthetized Edward Abbot on October 16, 1846, at Massachusetts General Hospital so that surgeon John Collins Warren could remove a large tumor on the man's jaw. James Young Simpson, a professor of obstetrics in Edinburgh, was one of the first to use ether in Great Britain.

The need for anesthesia was not, however, universally perceived to be necessary.[9] Some doctors were reluctant to use anesthesia because they felt its use increased blood loss during surgery and that it slowed the healing process afterwards. Some also held the opinion that the pain experienced by a patient during surgery without anesthesia would ward off the shock often induced by blood loss during the procedure. Other doctors held to the theory that pain during surgery was normal, and that surgery had to involve some amount of pain in order to be effective. This was the same type of misguided thinking that led some patients to believe that medicine had to taste disgusting in order for it to be effective.

After the introduction of anesthesia, surgery became more common because speed was no longer the main concern and doctors could take their time. The biggest boost to using anesthesia came during the Civil War when surgeons on the battlefield experienced the benefits both for themselves and for their patients when treating wounds without pain. Over 80,000 surgical operations were performed using anesthesia over the course of the war.

Nitrous Oxide

Nitrous oxide was discovered in 1772 by chemist Joseph Priestley in England, but he did not realize that the gas had anesthetic properties. In 1799, chemist Humphrey Davy, also in England, discovered that nitrous oxide induced a feeling of euphoria, relaxed the muscles, and made him laugh. Because of this property, he called it "laughing gas" and proposed that it might be used during surgery as an anesthetic to relieve pain.

Nitrous oxide was very short-acting, on the order of only a few minutes, so it was used primarily for brief, simple procedures such as the extraction of a decayed tooth.

Ether

Ether was formed by treating ethyl alcohol with sulfuric acid. The result was a clear, colorless liquid that was sweet-smelling and had anesthetic properties. In 1815, scientist Michael Faraday discovered that breathing ether fumes gave him a sense of euphoria.

The use of ether, however, had some disadvantages. One was that it was highly flammable and could even explode during an operation if any spark were present. Other drawbacks were that ether was difficult for the patient to take, was comparatively slow-acting, had a disagreeable smell, and caused increased coughing. In some ways, ether was more dangerous for the patient than chloroform because it initially acted to dilate blood vessels and promote bleeding if there was a laceration in the flesh, such as from a gunshot wound. As a result, the use of ether worsened shock and lowered blood pressure. The aftereffects were unpleasant and caused the patient to experience nausea, vomiting, and headache. Some surgeons, however, reported fewer deaths when using ether rather than chloroform.

Ether was administered by dropping the liquid onto a cloth placed over the patient's mouth and nose. Arthur Hertzler recalled the slow speed at which ether acted when he operated on one patient who required general anesthesia. He later wrote in his memoirs, "A local doctor gave the anesthetic. He dropped ether for a solid hour. At the end of this time he announced that the patient was ready. She asked, 'What did you say, doctor?' She had not even started to go to sleep."[10]

Chloroform

Chloroform was another substance commonly used for anesthesia. It was developed by American chemist Samuel Guthrie in New York, who distilled chloride of lime with alcohol in 1831 to produce chloric ether, later called chloroform. Scottish physician James Young Simpson used ether for obstetric cases but became unhappy with the weight of the ether bottles and concerned with the flammable properties of the material. So in January of 1847 he became the first to use chloroform in Edinburgh to relieve the pain of childbirth.[11]

The administration of chloroform to a patient was done mostly by guesswork, but it had to be given carefully. If the patient was overdosed he could die from respiratory collapse. Enough of the drug had to be administered to make the patient lose consciousness, then it was withdrawn gradually to allow a smooth recovery.

During the Civil War, chloroform was commonly used as an anesthetic with few complications. As more experience with anesthesia during battlefield surgery was gained, chloroform was used by army surgeons 76 percent of the time. Ether was used 14 percent of the time, and a combination of the two was used about 10 percent of the time. Even though chloroform was widely employed during the Civil War, surgeons in the field sometimes ran short and had to resort to surgery without anesthesia.

The technique for administering chloroform was to pour the liquid onto a cloth or napkin which was then placed over the patient's nose and mouth. The chloroform acted within about three minutes. Sometimes the patient was given whiskey, brandy, or some other liquor before the chloroform to produce a calming effect and help overcome the feeling of suffocation that often accompanied anesthesia.

The first stage of anesthesia was excitement, followed by delirium, struggling, muscle spasms, and attempts to rise up. Throat spasms could lead to breathing difficulties. Early anesthesia was restricted to this stage, which induced unconsciousness and reduced the severity of pain during the operation. This light level of anesthesia still required several burly assistants to hold the patient steady, while the surgeon operated at high speed. Because the patient thrashed around, even though unconscious, the common, but erroneous, perception was that many of the soldiers during the Civil War were not given anesthesia. It was not until the late 1800s, when the principles of anesthesia were better understood, that patients were put into what was called the second stage of anesthesia, which produced total unconsciousness and the relaxation of voluntary muscles.

The use of chloroform caused some embarrassment among doctors when anesthesia for obstetrical cases became more common in the early 1850s. As some women went under the influence of the anesthetic, they shouted obscenities and appeared to show signs of sexual excitement.

On the positive side, chloroform smelled pleasant and acted fast. It was pleasanter than ether for the patient to take, the recovery was quicker, and the aftereffects were less disagreeable. Chloroform was non-flammable, unlike ether, which could explode. This allowed the use of chloroform if candles or oil-lamps were used for lighting during an operation in a home or saloon. Ether fumes were too dangerous to use if a flame were present.

On the negative side, chloroform often caused vomiting, prostration, and increased excitement in the patient. Chloroform was not considered as safe as ether because its use could disrupt the action of the heart; chloroform was said to have caused five times as many deaths as ether. One example was a Mrs. Stump, who died in childbirth in Tombstone in 1884 when the doctor inadvertently gave her an overdose of chloroform.

Gunshot and Arrow Wounds

Life in the Old West was not the constant round of gunfights and Indian battles that are commonly depicted in motion pictures. However, fights between combatants armed with guns, and occasional skirmishes with hostile Indians, resulted in gunshot injuries and arrow wounds that were treated with surgical techniques by both civilian doctors and military surgeons. Lead bullets fired by a gunfighter's weapon in the Old West traveled at a low velocity, deformed on impact, became lodged in body tissues, and carried with them pieces of clothing and skin.

Wounds from gunshots and arrows were subject to the same types of infection as contemporary surgical procedures. Oliver Loving, for example, who, with Charles Goodnight, pioneered the Goodnight-Loving trail for bringing cattle from Texas to Colorado, was attacked by Comanche raiders on the open prairie of the dangerous Indian-infested country of northern Texas in 1867. He managed to escape but suffered wounds in the wrist and side. He went to the military hospital at Fort Sumner, New Mexico, for treatment but refused amputation of his arm until his partner Goodnight arrived. By the time Goodnight finally arrived, gangrene had set in, and Loving died that same night.

Gunshot wounds were typical after the shooting sprees that erupted as a result of too much drinking in a saloon. Wounded men were typically hit in the arm or leg by a soft lead bullet. The wound would probably become infected, and the man would probably lose that arm or leg, but the odds were about seven to one in favor of him recovering. The threat of infection was always present, and gangrene developed in about 20 percent of the cases. In Dodge City, on July 26, 1878, a shooting spree involving several cowboys resulted in a man named George Hoy receiving a bad wound in the arm. The assistant surgeon at nearby Fort Dodge amputated the arm in an attempt to save the man's life, but Hoy never recovered from the operation and died on August 21.

Some surgeons followed Lister's lead and used carbolic acid to clean their hands and instruments. Dr. George Goodfellow of Tombstone, Arizona, took great pains with disinfection and, by doing so, garnered an excellent reputation for saving patients with abdominal gunshot wounds.

Gunfights could start at the least provocation—often over a woman. "Teddy Blue" Abbott, a cowboy who rode the cattle trails of the West, recalled this story about a Texan whom he called George Hay:

> Hay was with a girl one night and the sheriff was stuck on this girl, and he came to the door and said: "Let me in or I'll kick the door in." George Hay said: "If you do I'll shoot you." And the sheriff went ahead and kicked it in, and George shot him and killed him. If he hadn't, the sheriff would have killed him, sure.[12]

Sometimes it took more than a single bullet to kill a gunfighter. This was the case during the gruesome revenge fight that took place in Medicine Lodge, Kansas, on June 19, 1873, between Arthur McCluskie and Hugh Anderson when they wounded each other several times. The shootout took place with a separation of about fifty feet between the two men. McCluskie was shot in the mouth, shoulder, and stomach. In spite of these wounds, McCluskie shot Anderson in the belly. When Anderson fell to the ground, McCluskie crawled over, with blood running from his various wounds, and killed Anderson with a stab wound in the side.

Not all gunshot wounds, however, were the result of gunfighters shooting each other. Many emigrants in wagon trains accidentally shot themselves, or others, in the leg or hand by keeping a gun at the ready that they were not experienced enough to handle. More deaths occurred in this manner on the Oregon Trail than those from Indian attacks.

Men who carried guns on purpose, such as lawmen and professional gunmen, were also prone to accidental injury, as evidenced by the following story about a man from Galeyville, Arizona. "While showing what an expert he was at twirling a six-shooter, Jim Johnson shot himself in the leg. Blood poisoning set in, and the doctor said amputation was necessary. But Jim wouldn't have it.... So Johnson saved his leg and lost his life."[13] In a similar instance, when a man in Clairmont, New Mexico, was demonstrating a fancy spin with his revolver in 1884, the gun accidentally discharged, neatly blowing off the thumb and the ends of three fingers from John Kelly, a former deputy sheriff, who was standing nearby.

Scalping by Indians was an unpleasant fate suffered by early settlers. Scalping did not always mean death and complete removal of the hair, and if attended to in time, the remnants of the scalp could sometimes be sewn back in place. Alcoholic Judge W.H. Baldwin (not a legal jurist, but a one-time judge of sheep at the Colorado territorial fair) was scalped by Indians in South America but survived with most of his hair. He also survived after being shot and badly wounded near Colorado Springs, Colorado, in 1868 by Arapaho Indians, who tried to scalp him again. When they realized that he had previously been scalped, they left him alone to die, probably due to superstitions about scalping him a second time. After surviving all this, Baldwin met an ignominious end when he stumbled into a shallow well at a slaughter house and drowned.

The lead bullets fired by early rifles and pistol were round, and were consequently called "balls." They tended to create relatively simple round puncture holes as they passed through tissue. Josiah "Doc" Scurlock, who rode with Billy the Kid in the Lincoln County cattle war, had his front teeth shot out in a gunfight. In spite of how gruesome this sounds, the bullet exited the back of his neck, luckily missing the spinal column and causing no serious damage.

That is not to say that these bullets were ineffective. A round ball made a wound that was much larger than the caliber of the weapon it was fired from. A .45 caliber slug had a terrible impact.

Later conical bullets tumbled end-over-end as they flew through the air, creating jagged, gaping wounds and massive injury to body tissue upon impact. These pointed projectiles often deformed as they plowed through flesh or struck a bone, creating jagged fragments of soft lead that further ripped the flesh apart inside a wound.

Bullets were extracted with various forceps and bullet clamps—often unwashed—or by specially-designed snares and metal scoops. A popular tool for extracting bullets was an instrument with a threaded tip on the end that was screwed into an embedded lead bullet, then carefully withdrawn through the hole in the flesh that the bullet had made when it entered.

One of the specialized instruments used for locating bullets in wounds was called the Nélaton Probe, named after its inventor, who was a French military surgeon. The device was a thin flexible wand about eight inches long, with a porcelain tip, that was inserted into the wound, along the bullet's pathway, to try and find the projectile. If the probe came into contact with something solid, the doctor assumed that it was the bullet, though it could just as well be a section of fractured bone. The probe had a rough surface at the end. If a hard object was encountered, the probe was rotated and then withdrawn. If the obstruction was a bullet, as opposed to bone, traces of lead would be found on the porcelain tip. These probes were criticized for causing additional damage to the tissues, but their use continued for decades.[14] At the time these devices were first utilized, probes were not sterilized; thus, they often carried additional infection deep into wounds.

The single most common cause of death from a gunshot wound was bleeding and the resultant loss of a large volume of blood. Obviously, if a bullet struck a vital organ, massive damage and internal bleeding would occur. But even a relatively minor wound in an arm or leg could continue to bleed and eventually kill the victim from shock due to loss of blood.

Many gunshot wounds were not immediately painful, as the body naturally anesthetized wounds as part of the process of shock. The pain came later, most of it after the wound became infected. Then large doses of opiates were needed. When "Rowdy Joe" Lowe had his shoot-out with Red Beard in Delano, Kansas, on October 27, 1873, he sent a load of buckshot into Beard's right arm and hip. Though not immediately fatal, Beard's wounds became infected, and he lingered for two weeks before he died.

The outcome of a gunfight was not good for a wounded participant. Doctors in small Western towns often operated on wounded patients under primitive conditions, with few antiseptics and sometimes without anesthetics. A man wounded in a gun battle might be treated by the light of a flickering candle or oil lamp in a saloon while lying on a pool table or card table. Surgical instruments were carried from patient to patient without the doctor washing or disinfecting them. The doctor often used his unwashed fingers to find and extract splinters of bone, the bullet in a wound, and pieces of clothing carried into the wound by the bullet.

In 1856, Dr. Thomas D. Hodges bet fifty dollars with a gambler that he could save the life of a wounded miner, Ezra Williams, who was shot in a saloon brawl. In a classic example of saloon surgery, Hodges operated on Williams while the patient was lying on a pool table. The locals pulled up their chairs to hold an overnight vigil with the doctor. Williams almost made it but died at dawn the next morning. More than losing a patient, who probably wouldn't have survived his wounds anyway, the doctor was concerned with losing his prestige as a surgeon.

Men suffering from gunshots or other serious wounds in remote parts of the Old West often died while being transported to help, jolting on a horse or lying in the back of a wagon on the way to a doctor in town. Ambulances for transporting the injured were essentially non-existent and were only available to the army. The civilian population had to make do with a wagon, a horse, or even a litter. Delays in transporting an injured man to medical treatment often proved fatal.

Even if participants in a gunfight sustained what only appeared to be minor wounds, infection that produced blood poisoning and gangrene were constant risks. Men wounded in a gunfight either lived or died according to their wounds, their individual constitutions, and a large amount of luck. The chances of survival for the wounded under these conditions were about 50 percent. For most of the wounded it was a case of let nature take its course.

One tragic double death that occurred as a result of a gunfight in December 1885 was that of Jack Saunders and William Bacon, who were partners in a brothel near Fort Fetterman in central Wyoming. The two men became involved in a dispute over money. Bacon drew his gun and shot Saunders in the stomach. Saunders, though fatally wounded, was able to draw his own gun and shoot Bacon in the throat. Saunders died two days later. Bacon survived, though with the bullet still firmly lodged in his throat. A Dr. Watkins came from Buffalo, Wyoming, to remove the bullet. Unfortunately, while the doctor was trying to remove the bullet, it slipped from his grasp and Bacon choked to death.

Being shot in the abdomen, referred to as being "gutshot," invariably damaged a vital organ and caused massive amounts of bleeding. Gunshot wounds that tore the stomach or small intestine were invariably fatal. Abdominal wounds that punctured the large intestine were not much better and were fatal about 90 percent of the time. The cause of death was either unchecked internal bleeding or the eventual onset of peritonitis as deadly bacterial organisms leaked into the belly cavity from a perforated gut. A wounded man might linger in agony for a day or two—or longer—with no hope of recovery.

If the victim recovered at all, which was extremely unlikely, he would require intensive amounts of nursing, as he would be unable to eat or drink. Dehydration, infection, and pain were inevitable. A victim would linger in agony for days or weeks before succumbing to infection.

On October 28, 1880, marshal Fred White of Tombstone, Arizona, tried to arrest William Graham (also known as Curly Bill Brocius) and some other cowboys who were shooting up the town. White ordered Graham to hand over his gun, and when White suddenly grabbed for the weapon, it discharged into White's stomach. The marshal suffered in agony for several days before he died.

Doctors treating gunshot wounds were sometimes threatened by a friend or relative to ensure that they did a good job. When Dr. Jerome Glick of Bannack, Montana, was called to treat a gunshot wound in the arm of Henry Plummer, the outlaw sheriff who was systematically robbing and terrorizing the local citizenry, he was threatened by the rest of Plummer's gang. Luckily for Glick, treatment was successful and Plummer recovered.

Soldiers

Due to the nature of their work in the West, solders fighting in the Indian Wars during the second half of the nineteenth century were exposed to the arrows and bullets of hostile opponents. Soldiers wounded in battle were told not to remove embedded arrows or to break off the shaft because the shaft indicated to the surgeon the direction that the arrowhead had traveled. An intact arrow in flesh was typically extracted by passing a wire loop down the shaft of the arrow and snaring the tapered head. The removal of an arrowhead that was embedded in a bone was more complex, and special clamps, snares, and forceps were used.

Soldiers were advised not to try to remove arrows by themselves; however, understandably, most of them did anyway. If a soldier was on patrol in a desolate and remote area of the West, far from his home fort, he might have no choice. Whether he did anything or not, the shaft of the arrow might break off after the arrowhead was embedded in the flesh, or the binding holding the arrowhead to the shaft might soften or loosen, thus leaving the arrowhead in the wound with no shaft sticking out. Arrowheads were usually bound loosely to the shaft by sinew, a fibrous part of animal tendons. After the arrow penetrated flesh, contact with blood or moist tissue often loosened the sinew, and the arrowhead separated from the shaft, making the head difficult to extract.

Some arrowheads were made of pieces of flint that were chipped to form a sharpened point. Nevertheless, these rough, crude weapons created jagged wounds and could penetrate deep into a vital organ. Other Indian arrowheads were cut from sheet metal, strap iron, or barrel hoops stolen from white settlers. These soft iron arrowheads often bent backwards when they hit a bone, causing the metal piece to become firmly lodged in the body like a fishhook. Extraction of this type of arrowhead, even by a surgeon, could cause further extensive tissue damage.

Soldiers wounded in battle might receive more injuries while lying helpless on the battlefield, or a severely wounded man might lie on the ground with bleeding wounds for hours before he could be rescued or treated. One word-of-mouth cure for bleeding wounds when far from help was to grind gunpowder into a fine consistency, apply it to the wound, and bind it up. A similar emergency treatment was to use the powered leaves and flowers of the goldenrod plant to stop bleeding. This was not original to the West but had been used for centuries to treat battlefield wounds.

CHAPTER NINE

The Hazards of Western Industry

Accidents associated with work have always been responsible for many deaths, injuries, and industrial illnesses. The same was true in the Old West. Many jobs were linked to specific injuries and illnesses, and various industrialized tasks were responsible for health problems in those who worked at them.

A common chronic ailment from the outdoor life and work was catarrh, which was a generic name for inflammation of the lungs and throat. The true cause could range from a respiratory infection to asthma or emphysema caused by dirty, dusty working conditions. Another generic complaint, particularly among those who worked in damp, cold conditions or who slept in tents or on the ground, was rheumatism. This group of complaints ranged from stiff and sore muscles to arthritis and degenerative muscular disease. Sleeping or working outside in rain or damp weather led to frequent colds and flu, which could then lead to pneumonia. Then, as now, influenza, also known as "the grippe," was widespread in winter.

Mountain Men and Trappers

The mountain men and trappers who first penetrated the West, searching for beaver pelts to sell to manufacturers of hats for the gentlemen of the East, found that they had to rely on their own ingenuity to survive in remote areas. The trapper had to overcome snow and cold, hunt his own food, live off the land, and eke out a precarious existence by himself or with a small group of fellow trappers.

Because of the mountain man's voluntary isolation from the rest of civilization, he was not as subject to catching contagious diseases, such as typhoid and yellow fever, as residents concentrated in the cities of the Northeast or the South. His health challenges were mainly accidents and wounds, or attacks by animals, such as bears or mountain lions. Other dangers were frostbite and the arrows of hostile Indians.

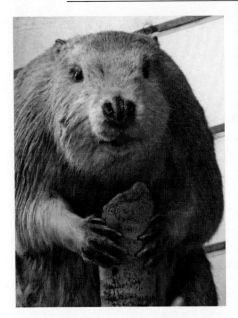

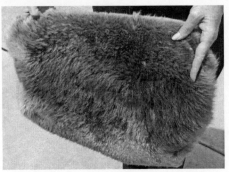

Mountain men and fur trappers inevitably suffered from rheumatism and arthritis from standing in cold mountain ponds and streams to trap for beaver. Prime pelts like this one (above) were a staple of commerce and were so valuable that they were nicknamed "hairy banknotes" (author's collection).

Most mountain men were of a solitary nature and used their own survival skills if they were injured or sick. On this basis, they either survived or they did not. The rugged frontiersman of the West knew how to set a broken bone, how to remove an embedded Indian arrow, and how to treat dysentery. Some trappers and traders married — or lived with — Indian women, who might treat them with basic nursing or use herbal remedies if they fell ill.

Trappers had to survive year-round in the hostile environment of the high mountains, where the weather was often unpredictable and where temperatures might fall well below freezing at any time of the year. During the height of the fall and spring beaver trapping seasons, when the fur was prime, a trapper's typical work day consisted of wading in icy mountain streams from dawn to dusk checking a string of from four to six traps, collecting and cleaning beaver pelts, and resetting the traps that had been sprung. Chronic arthritis brought on by standing and working for long hours in cold water, along with scars, bruises, and other physical handicaps from fighting Indians or wild animals, and muscular aches and pains from long hours of physical toil, made these men old before their time.

The lack of medical knowledge and care among mountain men made some cures quite primitive. In 1845, William Bent, one of the founders of the trading empire that surrounded Bent's Fort on the Arkansas River in Colorado, fell ill with what was probably diphtheria. As the disease progressed, his throat swelled to the point that he could no longer talk or swallow. In desperation, his Indian wife, Owl Woman, called in a Cheyenne medicine man. He looked into Bent's infected throat and decided on a "cure." He went outside the fort and collected several seedcases from sand-burr plants, which were covered in sharp thorns. The medicine man strung them onto a thread made of sinew and used a stick to push the burrs down Bent's throat. As he pulled the sinew and burrs back out, the sharp thorns scraped the putrid matter from Bent's throat. As barbaric as this treatment sounds, it worked. Afterwards, Bent was able to swallow soup, and in a couple of days he was up and about, on the way to a full recovery.

Prospectors and Miners

Miners were often the first pioneers in many parts of the West. For every cowboy, logger, or railroad worker, there were a hundred miners. Their environment and working conditions left them wide open to accidents and illnesses. Mumps, measles, smallpox, and other diseases accompanied prospectors and miners to the mountains, along with fevers, such as that due to typhus and others variously and unscientifically known as "lung fever," "bilious typhoid," and "ague fever."

Smallpox was common in mining camps as late as 1885. In 1880, records for the Storey County Hospital in Nevada listed thirty-six deaths from fever, thirty-five from pneumonia, and thirty-one from smallpox.

Many prospectors and miners became sick after arrival at the gold fields because of bad diet, poor preparation of food, sleeping on wet ground, and exposure to the cold, wet climate of high altitudes. A prospector often used his gold pan as an all-purpose utensil. As well as panning for gold with it, he washed his face in it, washed his dishes in it and, in a pinch, cooked in it and ate out of it. For the most part, miners' boarding houses were crowded, dirty, and poorly ventilated, thus contributing to the easy spread of disease among the men. Fleas and lice contributed to the unsanitary conditions of the camps. Trash and garbage were often strewn around as miners considered these to be temporary camps and hastily threw them together with minimal shacks for protection from the elements.

Dr. Jacob Stillman, a physician in the California gold fields, estimated that one miner in five died within six months of arrival. Records kept in Sacramento for the period 1851 to 1853 showed that out of a total of 1251 who died, 252 deaths were from fever, 237 from dysentery and diarrhea, 102 from cholera, and 125 from unknown causes. The latter figure confirms that physicians couldn't always determine what victims of illness actually died from.

Part of the problem lay with the inexact science of the diagnosis of disease. For example, in the early 1860s a mysterious disease named "mountain fever" appeared in the Colorado gold camps. It was characterized by abdominal pains, vomiting, constipation, and muscle spasms. Cases of the disease occurred periodically until the late 1880s when it just as mysteriously disappeared. Despite close investigation, the causes and source of the disease were never satisfactorily explained, though most physicians thought it was probably some variation of typhoid.

The Mining Environment

Miners and other workers in the outdoors suffered from aches and pains that were brought on by sleeping on wet ground, by winter's cold, by working in cold, damp environments, from carrying heavy loads, or through other stress on muscles. Miner's rheumatism, or "the rheumatiz" as they called it, was degenerative wear and tear of the joints from the strenuous labor of shoveling rock and performing the other physical tasks of mining. Today this would be considered some form of arthritis.

In this age of misdiagnosis, muscular aches and pains could have had several other causes. Inflamed joints could be a sign of rheumatic fever that eventually damaged the valves of the heart. Red, swollen, and painful joints might also be due to acute inflammation that was leading to blood poisoning.

Records for Leadville, Colorado, for 1879 showed that the commonest cause of death was rheumatism, followed by "crippled and maimed," with pneumonia as the third commonest cause. Pneumonia was a major killer in all the mountain camps. For those who caught pneumonia at high altitude, half the cases proved fatal.

Along with the miners, miners' wives and others living at high altitudes came down with pneumonia. Victims started out with a headache, tiredness, a loss of appetite, and a mild cough. As the disease advanced, the symptoms turned into chills, chest pains, a severe cough, and a high fever. At this stage of the disease, patients sometimes dropped dead. Others passed the crisis stage and eventually recovered. In the days before antibiotics, little could be done for the victim besides providing supportive care. The old standbys of bleeding, sweating, and a good dose of opium were tried, but these "cures" only served to weaken the patient. One of the few supportive measures that had a beneficial effect was to move the victim to a lower altitude where breathing was easier.

Much of the gold and silver mining in Colorado took place at altitudes higher than 9,000 feet, all the way up to the highest mines at 13,500 feet. Workers at these mines suffered from many of the symptoms of altitude sickness, such as headache, nausea, muscular weakness, stomach upsets, and sleeplessness. In winter, another danger at high altitudes was snow blindness

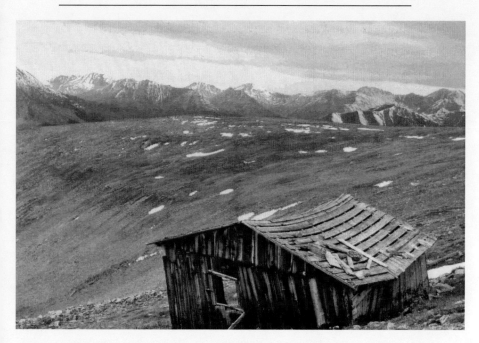

Many of the mines in the mountains were located on the bare slopes far above tree-line. Miners who lived and worked there frequently suffered from pneumonia, sunburn, and altitude sickness (author's collection).

from the intense sun reflecting off snowbanks. To protect their eyes, miners made primitive goggles, which consisted of a leather blindfold with narrow slits in them to reduce the amount of light. Eyeglasses with colored lenses were used, and charcoal was rubbed underneath the eyes to reduce the glare. The only treatment for snow-blindness was eye-drops and rest.

Another hazard of living at high altitudes in the mountains was the prevalence of lightning storms. The tallest object on a mountain peak or an open tundra meadow was often a man standing six feet or so above the surface of the ground. As a storm approached, hair stood on end and buzzed, skin tingled, metal objects clicked, and rocks developed an eerie purple glow as the air surrounding them became charged with electricity. Blue balls of electrical energy — St. Elmo's Fire — rolled along the ground. A miner or other person exposed on the top of a mountain had to heed these warnings and seek protection in the trees at a lower altitude before a bolt of lightning flashed down to relieve the electrical tension in the air. If lightning struck a man, it would kill him. At the Liberty Bell Mine, near Telluride, Colorado, a bolt of lightning struck the steel tracks for the ore carts that came out of the mine. In a freak accident, the electric charge traveled along the metal rails into the mine and killed three of the miners who were working underground.

Mining was hard, strenuous work. Many of the miners in Colorado lived to be only thirty-five or forty years of age because of the taxing working conditions. The high altitudes at many mines exposed miners to all the harsh conditions that went along with living in the high mountains. Fierce snowstorms in the winter, combined with heavy snow already on the ground, isolated many of the mines and trapped miners in their shacks for days on end, making it difficult to reach injured men in case they needed help.

One miner at the Humbolt Mine, located at an altitude of 12,600 feet in the mountains of southwest Colorado, set out in a blinding snowstorm for the town of Ouray, almost 5,000 feet below in the valley. As might be expected, he lost his way in the fierce storm and slipped off the steep trail, sliding almost 500 feet over ice, snow, and rocks into a narrow canyon. His body was seen — purely by chance — hours later by a group of passing miners. They found him unconscious, with a skull fracture and numerous cuts and bruises all over his body. They rescued him and took him down to the hospital in town, but he died of his injuries several days later.

Down in the Mines

The task of mining was a dangerous job. Miners were crushed, asphyxiated, buried, and blown up. Mining injuries resulted from blasting with dynamite, drills, hoists, tunnel collapses, rock falls, underground fires, and poison gas.

Each miner was required to "muck out" (load) the rock, debris, and ore that was blasted from the rock face during his shift. A typical requirement was to load eighteen one-ton ore cars during a ten-hour shift. The result was sore backs, aching arm muscles, and blisters and calluses all over the hands. At the end of a shift the men were tired and could easily make a mistake. Injuries resulted from being run over by an ore car or hit by falling rock. Rock dust was everywhere from drilling and shoveling broken rock into ore cars.

Men were injured riding in ore buckets, on cable tramways, and traveling up and down on mine hoists. They were crushed when they fell in shafts or were trapped in cave-ins. The timbering in mine shafts could collapse under them. Lumps of ore that had been blasted might remain hanging on a rock face by only the slightest hold and at the least jar could fall on an unsuspecting miner working below. In the Comstock mining district of Nevada there were 300 mining fatalities between 1865 and 1880. During the peak mining years, typically at least one serious mining accident occurred each day.

Early methods of drilling resulted in crippling injuries to fingers and hands. Hand drilling was accomplished by one of two methods. One was single jacking, where a miner held the drill bit in one hand and hit it with a small four-pound sledgehammer held in the other. The other method was double jacking, which required two miners. One held the drill bit and rotated it after each blow, while the other wielded a heavy eight or ten-pound sledgehammer with all his might. If the miner with the hammer slipped or misjudged his target in the dim light of the flickering candles, the miner holding the drill could suffer serious injury.

Later mechanized equipment used to drill holes in rock for dynamite was even more dangerous. Drilling machinery was taller than a man and was braced in place from the roof of the tunnel to the floor. The drills were powered by compressed air supplied through pipes from a large compressor located at the surface. Drill bits could become bound up, and the entire machine would kick back and hit the operator. For this reason, early rotary drills were called "widowmakers." Noise from the steel drill-bit grinding into rock was incredible in an enclosed space, and drill operators suffered deafness after only a short period of time on the job.

The first mechanized drilling was performed dry. That is to say, the drilling mechanism forced the steel bit into dry rock, creating a cloud of dust and rock chips as it did so. Miners considered rock dust to be merely an annoyance. But men breathing this perpetual cloud of rock dust soon con-

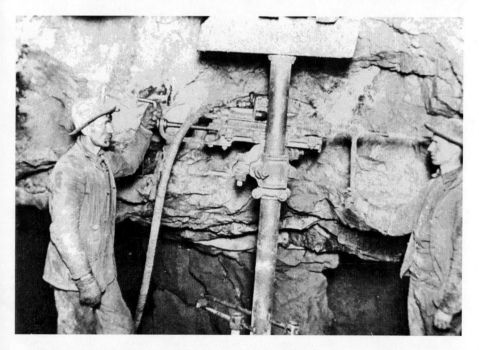

This type of rock drill was named the "widowmaker." These powerful drills, operated by compressed air, could kick back and seriously injure or kill the operator (Glenn Kinnaman, Colorado and Western History Collection).

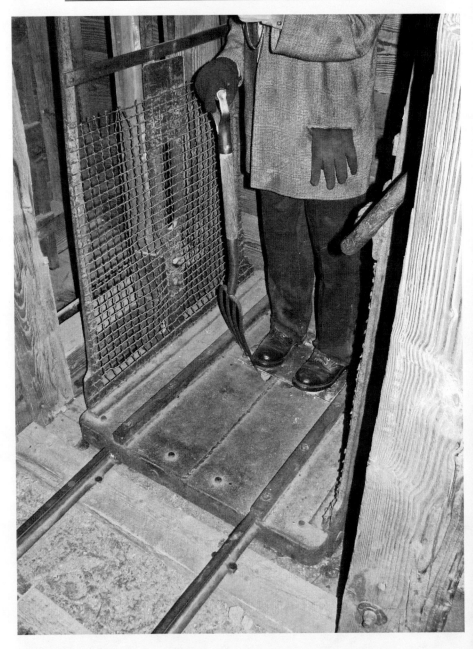

Hoist cars consisted of a simple steel frame with only partial protection on the sides, while the cage was lowered rapidly down a mine shaft. Injuries resulted from inadvertently sticking an arm or foot out of the open side while the car was in motion (author's collection).

tracted silicosis, a disease created when rock dust was inhaled into the lungs, where it irritated the pulmonary tissue, then scarred it. The scarring hardened the lungs so that they were not able to expand to draw sufficient oxygen into the bloodstream. The unfortunate victim was left choking and gasping for breath. After twenty years or so of working in the mines, a man could no longer work — or breathe. Some miners only lasted as few as three years before developing the disease. The progressive disease was called "miner's consumption," "miner's con," "callicosis," or "miner's phthisis."[1] This problem was alleviated by the introduction of hollow drills that sprayed water into the drill-hole and reduced the dust as the drill-bit rotated.

Cave-ins of shafts and tunnels that maimed and crushed miners were common.[2] During the early development of hard-rock mines, miners simply dug a hole down into the ground. As the shaft grew deeper, the ore and waste rock was hauled to the surface by a windlass operated either by hand or by a donkey or horse. As the mine grew progressively deeper, it was necessary to shore up the sides of the shaft with timber to prevent collapse. When the shaft was only twenty or thirty feet deep, the miners often did not bother to do this unless the surrounding rock crumbled easily. The result was that the sides of a shaft dug in loose rock or sandy soil could easily collapse and bury the miner working at the bottom. If the collar, the area around the shaft at the surface, was not reinforced, it could easily collapse and carry anyone standing at the edge down into the shaft.

As a mine grew deeper and the shaft reached hundreds, and even thousands, of feet into the ground, timbering solid enough to prevent collapse was essential. Timbering in mine shafts and tunnels had to be designed and constructed properly or it was unsafe and the tunnels subject to cave-in.

The steam-powered hoists that brought ore cars to the surface were subject to mechanical failure. Miners rode hoist cages up and down the shaft at the beginning and end of their shifts, often standing on top of the ore carts. The tiny cages had open sides, and an arm or leg protruding out of the side could be sheared off in an instant while the cage was moving. Any defect or weakness in the hoist cable and it would give way, the cage plummeting to the bottom of the shaft, carrying the miners with it. George Witcher was killed in this manner in a mine in the Tombstone silver mining district in 1882 when a cable broke and the cage he was riding in dropped like a rock to the bottom of the shaft.

Conversely, ascending in a cage was also dangerous. The engineer running the hoist machinery was supposed to apply the brakes when the cage was approaching the surface and bring it to a smooth stop at the loading station. Occasionally, however, mechanical or operator failure occurred, and the cage was pulled at full speed up into the head-frame, killing the men.

Another hazard faced by miners was the extremely acidic water found

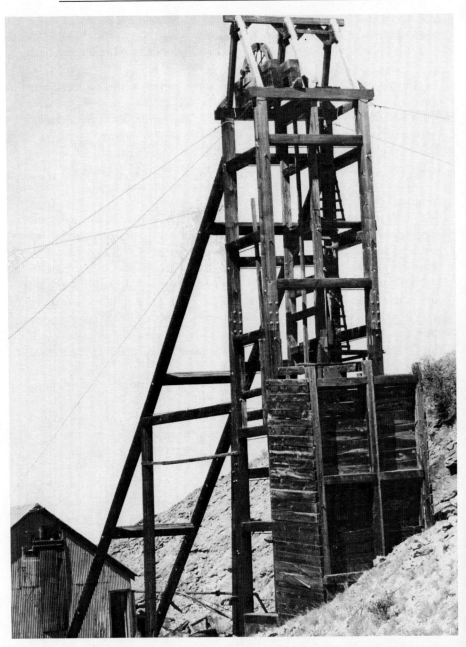

Hoist cars were raised and lowered from a headframe built over the mine shaft. If the operator was not careful, the cage could be accidentally pulled over the top of the hoist wheel, injuring or killing those riding in the cage (Glenn Kinnaman, Colorado and Western History Collection).

in some gold and silver mines. Metal parts on pumps, rails, and ore cars were quickly eaten away. In the Red Mountain mining district of Colorado a metal shovel or similar tool left accidentally in contact with the mine water overnight would have large holes eaten in it by morning due to a high content of sulfuric acid in the water seeping from the walls. The acidic water ate away at the men's clothing and skin, and the acrid fumes irritated the lungs.

Poisonous water also made its way to the surface, and local water supplies in mining camps were often contaminated with high levels of lead, arsenic, and copper that had leached from the mines due to the acid water. One humorist in Virginia City, Nevada, said that the poisonous water there could be purified by adding half a drinking glass full of whiskey to a spoonful of water in order to make it palatable for drinking.

Early mines had no provisions for underground toilet facilities. As a result, old workings were used for bathrooms, and miners urinated and defecated wherever they could find an abandoned tunnel. This fetid working atmosphere was augmented by droppings from mules that worked underground to pull the ore cars before the development of tram engines powered by compressed air. Water polluted by human and animal waste often leaked into lower levels of the mine or into the local groundwater. The larger mines eventually used a honeywagon, a small enclosed tank car with a toilet seat on top that was rolled along the same tracks as the ore cars.

The mines around Virginia City, Nevada, were situated on top of a hydrothermal area. Many mines in the Comstock mining district were deep, and as the depth grew, the working temperatures increased — often to above 100° F. The temperature at the 3,000-foot level of the Yellow Jacket Mine was one of the highest, producing working conditions that reached an incredible 167° F. Water that permeated through the ground became boiling hot, and if a miner accidentally dug into an underground water pocket, he could be scalded to death by the resulting geyser of hot water spraying out over him. Men drank literally gallons of water on each shift and chewed on ice to try and stay cool enough to work. Even these precautions might not be enough, and men at the deepest levels of the mine occasionally died from heat prostration. As well as contending with the heat, the men worked in air that was poor and stagnant, and laden with dust and noxious fumes that led to respiratory diseases.

An unseen danger in the mines was poisonous gases. The gas might be inert, such as carbon dioxide, and would displace all the breathable air in a pocket. Miners inhaling it would pass out and, if not rescued within two or three minutes, would suffocate from lack of oxygen. Pockets of poisonous hydrogen sulfide would kill quickly in a similar manner.

Another dangerous gas encountered in many mines was methane gas. Methane was highly explosive, and a miner digging into a rock face containing methane, or passing into a stagnant pocket of methane with a lighted candle or the open flame of a carbide lamp, would not live to tell the tale. Methane (also called "marsh gas" or "fire damp") was common in the coal mines of both the East and the West.

Fires underground were deadly and a particularly nasty way to die. As smoldering fires grew in intensity, the heat and fumes overcame many of the men. Others collapsed and died as the fire sucked all the available oxygen out of the air. Along with the smoke that resulted from burning material, a fire in a mine created carbon monoxide, the same deadly gas generated in automobile exhaust fumes and improperly vented furnaces. Carbon monoxide inhibits the oxygen-carrying capacity of the blood and basically suffocates the victim. One such fire started on April 7, 1869, at the 800-foot level of the Yellow Jacket Mine, probably from a miner's candle that was left behind unnoticed at the end of a shift and ignited one of the support timbers. Smoke and poisonous gases roared through the underground workings and killed fifteen miners in a nearby tunnel.

Worse than that was the fire at the Crown Point Mine in the same district. Miners were being lowered to work at various levels in the mine when they encountered smoke and poisonous gas. The hoist operator, not realizing what was happening underground, continued to lower the cage into the deadly atmosphere. When the horrible situation was discovered, a few of the miners were raised to safety. Dense black smoke soon billowed through interconnecting tunnels to the neighboring Kentuck, Yellow Jacket, and Crown Point mines. Before the fire was subdued, forty-five miners had died. Some were found at the bottom of shafts where they had plunged to their deaths, probably running blindly through unlighted tunnels, trying to find an escape route or a hoist cage that was not there.

Dynamite

Dynamite used for blasting out rock in the mines was a tricky substance to handle and was a common source of accidents. Miners had to be experienced in its properties to deal with it safely.

The first useful explosive in the mines was black powder, a mixture of saltpeter, potassium nitrate, and charcoal that was also used in contemporary revolver and rifle cartridges. In 1867, chemist Alfred Nobel in Sweden developed dynamite, a far more powerful explosive agent. Dynamite was based on nitroglycerin, an explosive substance developed in 1847, but which was so powerful and unstable that it was not suitable for use in its pure liquid form. To make it useable, nitroglycerin was combined with an inert substance, such as wood flour, sawdust, or chalk. The mixture, formed into sticks about eight inches long and an inch or so in diameter, then wrapped in paraffined paper, was called dynamite. Dynamite was also nicknamed "giant powder."

Unlike nitroglycerin, a stick of dynamite was very stable and had to be ignited by either a sharp blow or an electrical spark. The sharp blow was provided by a percussion cap, a short cylindrical device, about two inches long and a half-inch in diameter, filled with fulminate of mercury, a highly unstable substance.[3] Sparks from a burning fuse ignited the percussion cap, which then exploded and, in turn, caused the stick of dynamite to explode.

The procedure for blasting out gold and silver ore was to drill a hole in the rock face to be broken up. When the hole was about three or four feet deep, a metal spoon was used to clean out the debris. A percussion cap with a fuse was attached to a stick of dynamite, and the combination was carefully packed into the hole with a wooden rod (to prevent sparks from igniting the dynamite). When all the dynamite charges were ready, the fuse was lit and the explosives did the rest. Multiple sticks of dynamite might be used in a single hole when blasting a rock face at the end of a mine tunnel. Blasting was typically done at the end of a shift so that there was time for the dust to settle before the next shift of miners arrived to muck out the broken debris at the rock face.

In practice, a pattern of holes, usually in a circle, was drilled in the rock face to be blasted out, and a stick of dynamite was forced into each hole. Here was the first danger. If a stick of dynamite had become unstable, the pressure of tamping it into place could be enough to cause it to explode, firing the tamping rod out of the hole like an arrow through the miner using it.

In one particularly gruesome accident, three men, named Robinson, Maloney, and Burns, were loading dynamite into the ore face of a tunnel as their shift ended. Something — perhaps a spark of static electricity — set off the charge prematurely while the men were still in front of the drill holes. Robinson was decapitated and his chest blown open. Maloney's head was hit by flying rock, which fractured his skull and exposed his brain. Burns was luckier. He was hit in the face by splinters of rock. Though the bodies of the other two shielded Burns from much of the explosion, he spent the next six months in a hospital, though he eventually recovered from his injuries. A similar blast killed William Alexander, an old prospector at a mine in Tombstone, who was fatally injured in 1880 when dynamite exploded prematurely.

Each dynamite stick in the rock face to be blasted had a different length of fuse attached. Because of their dangling appearance, miners nicknamed the fuses "rat-tails." The fuse lengths were distributed so that each dynamite stick was set to explode at a slightly different time, in sequence. The miner in charge of setting off the blast counted the number of explosions, which told him that all the dynamite sticks had exploded. Occasionally one would not explode, resulting in a potentially lethal situation. An unexplored stick had to be carefully removed from its hole in the rock so that it could not explode unexpectedly while the loose rock was being loaded into ore carts, or if a miner struck it with a pick or shovel.

Removing unexploded dynamite was an extremely dangerous process because any stick that had not exploded was probably defective and could explode without warning. A missed shot might go off while it was being pried out with a tool during the removal process. Typical of the results was what happened at the Contact Mine in the central Colorado mountains when a miner named John Broll was attempting to remove an unexploded stick of dynamite from a drill-hole. Even though Broll was a careful and experienced miner, the charge blew up, killing him instantly. The corpse's left leg was shattered in three places, both hands were mangled, the back was broken, and Broll's face was peppered with small chips of rock as if from a shotgun.

Human errors could also occur. A distracted miner might miscount the number of explosions, leaving one unexploded round unaccounted for. Or he might have mistakenly packed two charges of dynamite into the same hole.

When dry and cool, dynamite was safe and stable. When temperatures fluctuated, however, it could be deadly. When dynamite became hot, it "sweated" drops of nitroglycerin that accumulated on the surface of the dynamite stick. Careless handling of the stick could cause the dynamite to explode prematurely and injure whoever was handling it, along with anyone nearby. If this occurred to a stick in a box of dynamite, sympathetic detonation occurred, and the resulting explosion of the whole box was disastrous.

Conversely, very low temperatures also caused problems. When dynamite froze in the sub-zero winter temperatures of the mountains it would not explode. To make it useable again, miners took the sticks into their cabins to thaw and held them near the stove or fireplace, or placed them in the oven. When the dynamite warmed, it became extremely unstable and was liable to explode at the slightest touch. The correct way to thaw dynamite was to use a warmer, which was a metal box filled with warm water. The

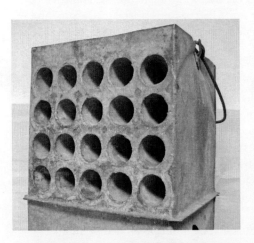

This metal warming box prevented the explosions that commonly occurred when frozen dynamite was thawed rapidly on a stove. A stick of dynamite was placed in each of these holes, and warm water was poured into the top of the tin box to slowly thaw each one (author's collection).

dynamite sticks were placed inside pipes that went from side to side in the outside of the box to allow warming while keeping the dynamite dry.

Typical of the results of incorrect warming was what happened to Billy Mayer in his cabin near the Virginius Mine, which was located at 12,200 feet in the San Juan Mountains of southwest Colorado. As he was thawing dynamite on the stove in his cabin, eight of the sticks exploded without warning. The stove shot through the roof of the demolished cabin like a rocket. Mayer was blown in a bloody heap under one of the bunks.

Mayer's partner, who received only slight injuries in the explosion, started off to the nearby Terrible Mine for help. The winter's accumulation of snow at 12,000 feet was so deep that it took the man seven-and-a-half hours to struggle a distance of one mile to the other mine. Four of the miners from the Terrible started back to Mayer's cabin wearing snowshoes, so they were able to make better time.[4] They strapped Mayer onto a makeshift sled and started for the nearest small settlement, Sneffels, which was three miles away. Four more men volunteered to come up to the Terrible from

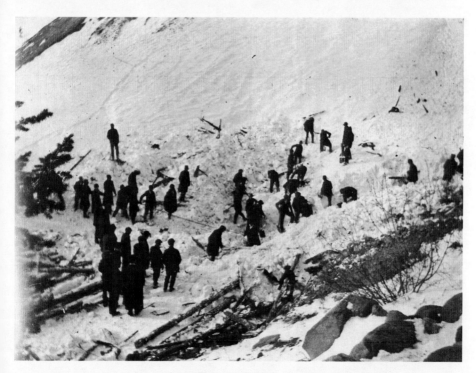

Snowslides were common and deadly in winter in the mountains. Workers here are digging for the bodies of ten Italian miners who were buried by a snowslide at the Seven-Thirty Mine on the steep slopes of Brown Gulch above Silver Plume, Colorado (Special Collections, Tutt Library, Colorado College, Colorado Springs).

town, seven miles further on, to help transport the injured man down to the nearest hospital. By now it was growing dark and a snowstorm had started.

The four relief men never showed up, so the original rescuers, already exhausted from struggling through the deep snow, had to take Mayer on down to the hospital. When the four miners returned to the Terrible Mine the next day, they noticed evidence of a fresh snowslide beside the trail. Looking closer, they found the missing rescuers from town buried in the snow, marked only by a single frozen hand protruding above the site of the snowslide.

In winter, miners sometimes carried sticks of dynamite in their pocket, in their boot, or strapped to their leg under their pants. The idea was that their body heat kept the sticks from freezing on the way to work. If the dynamite should explode, however, the consequences were fatal.

The blasting caps used to set off the dynamite were powerful explosive devices and could be dangerous. Like dynamite, blasting caps were commonly carried in a miner's pocket for easy access when required. By their nature, a sharp blow to the pocket or a faulty cap could result in a severe leg or groin injury. Missing fingers and hands from blasting cap explosions were common.[5]

A lesser, but nonetheless common, hazard of dynamite was its toxic effect on humans. Miners who handled dynamite frequently suffered from what was called "powder headache." In extreme cases of exposure, nausea, vomiting, and muscle twitching were present. The cause was the nitroglycerin in the dynamite, the same substance that was used medicinally in small doses to dilate blood vessels for the relief of pain, such as in heart disease (*angina pectoris*). Continued exposure to the nitroglycerin in dynamite, coupled with poor ventilation in the mines, produced chronic pounding headaches, low blood pressure, and bloodshot eyes.

Dynamite found general use not only in the mines but elsewhere in the West for blasting. Gilbert Lathrop, a railroad engineer, remembered the results when several tons of dynamite that were stored in a railroad storehouse in Colorado exploded:

Blasting caps, fired by a fuse or an electric spark, jolted dynamite sticks to make them explode (author's collection).

One night the giant powder let loose. Every windowpane in Chama was shattered. Tools, block and tackle, canned foodstuffs, and all kinds of railroad equipment were blown over the surrounding hills. A pit large enough to hold a good-sized house was left where the building had stood.[6]

Mills and Smelters

Freighters drove ore wagons between the mines and mills. They could be injured in roll-overs, swept away by avalanches or flooded rivers, or killed if their wagon drove off a narrow mountain road. Unloading ore to be processed from a tram car into the ore chutes at the mill could result in crushing injuries to hands and feet from the ore car, falling rock, or the mill equipment. Occasionally a careless worker fell into one of the ore chutes and was crushed to death either by falling rock or the heavy machinery used to reduce large chunks of rock to a suitable size for processing.

Work for the men in the mills and smelters that reduced gold and silver ore to precious metal was extremely dangerous. Mill workers were subjected to dust from milling, noise that deafened them, and machinery that could crush them instantly. Smelters were filled with toxic fumes from chemicals and roasting ores.

Ore was crushed to a fine consistency for concentration and processing by a row of heavy iron stamps, which were essentially huge iron hammers weighing several hundred pounds that were raised by a rotating cam and allowed to fall back down by gravity to crush the ore. A small mill might contain eight or sixteen stamps. Large mills used sixty to a hundred stamps.

One by-product of the stamp mill was a continual deafening, pounding, roaring noise that hung over the mill and the nearby town. Residents learned to mentally tune out the noise and knew that it meant that all was well. Miners knew that a serious accident or other major trouble had occurred at the mill if the stamps shut down and there was an unaccustomed absence of noise.

In Bodie, California, the Standard Mill was in full operation twenty-four hours a day, and the stamps were never shut down. Damaged stamps had to be repaired while the mill was in operation. To do this the damaged stamp was secured in a raised position by wooden blocks so that the rotating cam did not operate it while it was being repaired. The other stamps continued to pound the ore fed underneath them. One slip and the men doing the repair could lose a finger, hand, foot, or worse.

Mills and smelters for ore reduction used highly toxic chemicals, such as mercury and cyanide. Long-term exposure to these poisonous materials caused various health problems and premature death in workers.

Early reduction of free gold was performed by washing the gold ore over quicksilver (mercury) in a process called amalgamation.[7] Mercury had a strong affinity for gold and trapped the gold dust or flakes of gold passing

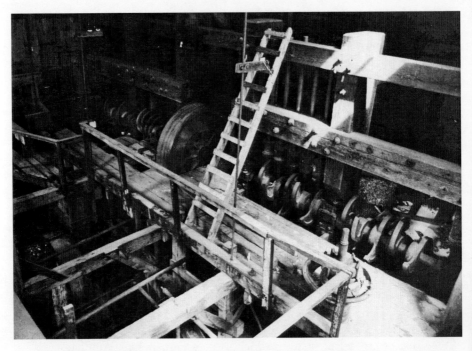

Ore processing machinery, such as these stamps at a stamp mill, was extremely dangerous and could quickly crush a hand, foot, or an entire body if a mill worker was not very careful (author's collection).

over it. The resulting gold-mercury mixture was heated to vaporize and drive off the mercury, leaving a concentrate of pure gold. The mercury fumes were trapped and cooled, and the liquid mercury collected for re-use. Though effective, this procedure was extremely dangerous because mercury fumes hung over the entire processing area and eventually poisoned the workers. Mercury fumes produced the same symptoms as mercury and calomel when used as a medicine. The men suffered from uncontrollable drooling and shaking, and loss of memory; their teeth fell out, their internal systems were upset, and they eventually went insane from brain decay.

Another process for extracting pure gold from waste rock involved bubbling chlorine gas through a sludge of gold-bearing ore. As in the mercury process, this volatile chlorine gas escaped into the air and affected the workers. Chlorine gas was so poisonous that it was used as an agent of chemical warfare in Europe during World War I. The gas scarred the lungs, and killed or maimed tens of thousands of troops in trench warfare in France, and left hundreds of thousands with inflamed lungs. A later, more advanced process treated gold ore with sodium cyanide, another highly toxic compound, to leach out gold particles into solution for reclaiming.[8]

Smelters involved a series of deadly health problems for mine and mill workers. The smelting process for gold and silver ores was basically a roasting process that heated the ore to very high temperatures to drive off undesired volatile components, such as sulfur, and concentrate the precious metals. The by-product was a nauseating, thick, oily smoke that hung over mill towns and caused various lung ailments among workers and the general population. Smelting towns, such as Blackhawk and Leadville in Colorado, and Butte in Montana, had dense clouds of arsenic, lead, and soot hanging over them. Leadville had over a dozen smelters by 1880 whose output covered the entire town with a dense pall of toxic yellow and black smoke. Butte, which was a large center for copper smelting, sent fumes of arsenic, sulfur, and copper into the air.

Other chemical hazards were present in gold and silver mining. Leadville, for example, had a high incidence of lead poisoning both in the mines and at the local smelters. Between 1880 and 1882, St. Vincent's Hospital in Leadville recorded treating 162 miners and 605 smelter workers for lead poisoning.

Cowboys

Though the image from motion pictures is that cowboys were always shooting each other and patching up gunshot wounds, that was not the reality. Cowboys were not professional gunfighters, and bullet wounds were rare. Many cattle bosses would not allow cowboys to carry guns on the trail. Hunting for venison or warding off the occasional Indian attack were the only times they carried firearms. Even rifles were typically banned to prevent them from catching on bushes and brush (and so throw the rider), and to prevent saddle sores on his horse from the extra weight. More likely than a gunfight was an accidental bullet wound from a carelessly handled revolver.

The health problems suffered by cowboys were primarily physical injuries resulting from working with horses and cattle. Cowboys were injured or died after being caught under stampeding cattle and buffalo herds. Sleeping on the ground in wet and cold weather led to arthritis and aching joints. A surprising number drowned while driving their herd across river crossings. Horses and riders could be gored by nervous or angry cattle, or could be trampled during a stampede. Cowboys were likely to be thrown or fall from their horse during a routine work day and break an arm or shoulder. Sometimes a boot would catch in the stirrup, and the unfortunate rider was dragged over rocks, cactus, and bushes, resulting in bruises and broken bones (and sometimes in death). Cowboy boots were made with slanting heels to prevent them from catching in the stirrup, but they didn't always release. Sprains,

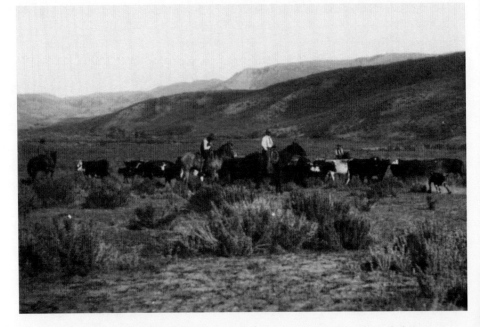

Cowboys at work were subject to sprains, bruises, broken bones, snakebites, gunshots, and even being gored or crushed to death during a stampede (Glenn Kinnaman, Colorado and Western History Collection).

fractures, and dislocations were common. Other injuries resulted from wagons turning over or running over men. Further dangers were burns during branding and being struck by lightning on the open prairie.

There were few old cowboys. Most cowboys were young and single, between eighteen and twenty-eight years of age, with the typical age being around twenty-four. A cowboy was old at age thirty, and most men quit after about ten or fifteen years on the job. Riding the range was a job for young men who had the strength and stamina for a hard physical life.[9]

Cowboys, and others who spent long hours in the saddle, were subject to blisters and saddle sores in delicate areas. A lack of vitamin C and the onset of scurvy, due to a poor diet on the trail, led to bleeding sores on the buttocks that did not heal until the scurvy was resolved. A more embarrassing complaint was temporary sterility among cowboys, cavalry soldiers, and others on horseback for long periods of time due to constant bouncing in the saddle.

One of the afflictions that plagued cowboys was a nasty type of dermatitis named "prairie itch." Though never satisfactorily explained, it was probably a type of scabies, a highly communicable disease caused by a female mite, *Sarcoptes scabiei*, called the "itch mite," that burrowed under the skin and laid its eggs. Cowboys who had "the itch" broke out in an irritating rash between the fingers, on the chest, around the genitals, and on the inner thighs. One cure was to sponge bichloride of mercury in alcohol on the skin.

As it was for the miners, breathing dust raised by the herd during a trail drive was a hazard to the lungs. Cowboy "Teddy Blue" Abbott recalled this about the men who rode at the back of the herd: "They would go to the water barrel at the end of the day and rinse their mouths and cough and spit and bring up that black stuff out of their throats. But you couldn't get it up out of your lungs."[10]

Out on the trail or on a cattle roundup far from the ranch-house, cowboys were a long distance from professional medical help in case of injury. The trail boss may have had some rudimentary experience in first aid and splinting broken bones, but often the closest medical care was the cook, who might carry some bandages and a few medicines in the chuck wagon. Serious illness, such as a snakebite or appendicitis, meant that the unfortunate cowboy had to tough it out on the trail. The victim might be lucky if the herd was relatively near to a town with a doctor. Usually, however, it was not, because the trail boss tried to pick his route away from towns and the temptations of whiskey and women that could interrupt the progress of the drive.

Snakebite was an ever-present problem on the Great Plains and in the Southwest. One frontier remedy for rattlesnake bite was to drink between a pint and a quart of whiskey. Besides dulling the pain (and obviously the senses), which may have made this a popular remedy, this "medicine" was said to neutralize the poison and effect a cure. Modern medicine does not favor alcohol after a snakebite because alcohol dilates the blood vessels of the skin and promotes absorption of the venom. A more positive folk cure was to bathe the snakebite in gunpowder mixed with vinegar. One later medical treatment was to treat the bite by cauterizing it with silver nitrate — then administering whiskey to the patient.

Rabies (hydrophobia) was a concern in the Old West, from bites by both domestic dogs and cats, and by wild animals that carried rabies, such as skunks, bobcats, coyotes, foxes, and bats. Rabies was certainly a problem to be reckoned with. Once contracted, the disease was incurable, and the victim died an agonizing death. Victims went into a violent rage and started frothing at the mouth before they sank into a coma and died. Occasionally, horses and other domestic livestock could become infected from the bite of a rabid animal and expose people to the rabies virus.

One of the duties of a town marshal on the frontier was to hunt down and shoot wild dogs in order to prevent danger from rabies. Wild Bill Hickok was paid fifty cents for every unlicensed dog that he shot while he was town marshal of Abilene in the 1870s. In spite of constant fears, Colorado's first reported case of rabies did not occur until 1899.

Sunstroke

In the deserts of the Southwest and on the Great Plains during the summer months, sunstroke (heatstroke) was common among men who worked outside under the broiling sun. The combination of overheating and dehydration shut down the body's cooling mechanism. Sweating stopped, and the victim became disoriented and fell into a coma. Body temperature rose rapidly above 105° F — even up to 112° F — and the victim broiled to death internally. If caught and treated in time, the condition could be reversed by cooling and re-hydrating the victim. If not, convulsions and death occurred.

Edward Dorris, a stagecoach driver for Barlow and Sanderson, was one of the unfortunate ones. He died at Bent's Fort on July 21, 1865, probably from sunstroke brought on by the heat of mid-summer and the harsh conditions along the Santa Fe Trail. He was only thirty-one years of age.

Frostbite

Cold weather brought a different set of dangerous conditions to residents of the Old West. In Wyoming temperatures could drop to -25° F to -40° F. In Montana they routinely dropped to -40° F. Cowboys, soldiers, railroad men, and other outdoor workers in these extreme temperatures were prone to the rapid onset of frostbite, which could cause a loss of fingers, toes, hands, or feet. During conditions of severe cold, ice crystals formed in the flesh, causing the skin to turn white and waxy, and the affected body parts to become as hard as wood. After the flesh froze, gangrene might set in, and amputation of fingers and toes was the only treatment.

Frostbite was a serious consideration on the Great Plains in winter, in the mining camps of the high mountain, and at high latitudes. As well as suffering from dysentery and scurvy, men in the gold rushes to Alaska and the Yukon were plagued by frostbite. The men who "wintered over" in the wilds to try and dig their fortunes out of the frozen ground braved sub-zero temperatures. At times the temperature dropped so low that even whiskey froze inside cabins, and metal tools fractured in the cold. The men suffered frozen fingers and toes that had to be thawed out over a stove in a drafty cabin. During the first year that William Ballou lived in the Yukon, seven of his friends froze to death. Another friend died during an operation to amputate both legs after they froze in a deadly spell of cold weather.

One new arrival in St. Michael, the port at the mouth of the Yukon River that served as the starting point for the water journey to the gold fields at Dawson, recalled seeing a man with no feet being carried on board ship on a friend's back. The man had been part of the gold rush at Dawson, but had neglected to provide himself with suitable footgear. Frostbite and gangrene set in, and the man's feet had been amputated after they froze.

Soldiers

Many soldiers suffered from chronic minor illnesses due to unhealthy living conditions in the outdoors, along with a poor diet. A common complaint was catarrh, an inclusive term for inflammation of the lungs and throat, perhaps brought on by asthma and emphysema from sleeping on the ground or in damp buildings. Soldiers in the field commonly slept on bare ground in all weather, often in wet clothing at the end of a rainy or snowy day. Living and sleeping for days at a time in the field in wet weather created a high incidence of arthritic complaints among the men. Wet clothes could rapidly turn a common cold into pneumonia and prove deadly. A frequent complaint was rheumatism, another generic term that included soreness and stiffness of the joints due to age, arthritis, previous muscle damage, or other conditions.

Due to the nature of their work, obviously, soldiers were subject to injuries during battles with hostile Indians. Gunshots, arrow wounds, or fragments of metal from exploding cannon shells were all severe hazards during battles. In addition, being thrown from a cavalry horse or crushed under the wheels of a supply wagon or military ambulance were a real possibility.

The standard cavalry saddle, the McClellan saddle, was hard and unpadded. The design was intended to save weight and prevent saddle-sores from developing on the horse's back, rather than for the comfort of the trooper. The disadvantage for the rider was that long hours spent in the saddle made hemorrhoids a common affliction for cavalry troopers, along with saddle-sores and blisters. Being unable to ride properly could affect the fighting performance of a cavalryman, and, if serious enough, could even affect his continued career.

Wounds sustained during an Indian fight might prove fatal in short order due to loss of blood or shock, or might turn fatal later due to the complications of surgery or subsequent infection and blood poisoning. Wounded soldiers might succumb to their wounds during the process of being transported from the battlefield back to their post. Battlefield wounds frequently became infested with flies and maggots.

Estimates showed that approximately 12 percent of the soldiers who served in winter on the northern Plains suffered from frostbite. In spite of precautions, some soldiers on winter campaigns simply froze to death. The first roll call of the morning often showed that some of the men had not made it through the night. During the bone-chilling winter Indian campaigns on the Great Plains, the first chore in the morning was a head-count to see if any of the soldiers had frozen to death during the night. One visitor to Fort Dodge, Kansas, was told that seventy amputations of limbs among the soldiers had been necessary during the preceding winter.

Railroad Accidents

Train crashes, derailments, explosions, and other railroad accidents made life for railroad workers very hazardous. Being burned by a hot firebox, scalded by steam escaping from the boiler, or slipping and losing a leg under a train were potential hazards that they faced every day. Estimates indicated that a man who chose to work for the railroads as a career had a 20 percent chance of being killed at work. Statistics for the year 1900 show that 7,865 men were killed in railroad accidents, and more than 50,000 were injured.

Aaron Harrison was an engineer for the Southern Pacific in Tucson, Arizona, when his engine was in a wreck near Rillito in 1888. He was scalded by steam escaping from the wrecked boiler and died from his injuries several days later. The boiler on Engine No. 35 on the Colorado Midland Railway exploded with such violence on August 6, 1896, that the engine virtually disintegrated and metal parts were blown several hundred feet in all directions.

Loose rails, rail-bed washouts, and overheating of axle boxes were common causes of train wrecks. Inspection of the Union Pacific's track shortly after the completion of the transcontinental railroad showed that bridges were unsafe, tunnels were too narrow, the railbed was often improperly leveled and ballasted, and some of the rails were mis-aligned.

Engineers and firemen quickly learned when to "unload," or jump from a train (often called "joining the birds"), when a wreck threatened. If they stayed with their engine they could easily be killed by the impact, or by steam and hot metal fragments if the boiler exploded. Gilbert Lathrop described an unexpected train wreck where this happened:

> The little consolidated rambled along in lively style until she came to a short, wooden trestle. When she was about to the center of it there came a crash, followed by a splintering of wood and a cloud of steam. The engineer and his fireman leaped to safety. But the section foreman [who was riding in the cab at the time] was not so lucky. He was crushed to death under the boiler.[11]

In another railroad accident on Marshall Pass in the Colorado Rocky Mountains, the brakes failed on a coal train going down the pass, and the engine piled up on a curve. The engineer, the fireman, and one of the brakemen were killed. The two other brakemen were seriously injured. Only the conductor survived without injuries.

The following incident, which occurred in 1882 on the Denver, South Park and Pacific Railway, was typical. As reported in the *Pitkin Review*:

> Yesterday afternoon an accident occurred on the above road at a point between Woodstock and the U [a hairpin turn], by which several parties

were more or less injured by jumping from the train when at full speed. It appears that the train was running at a rapid rate, and the engineer applied the air brakes, when something gave way, and he lost control of his engine and it ran away.... In the meantime several parties jumped from the train and were injured.[12]

Passengers were not immune from injury. Another paper had a different view of the same accident, as reported by the superintendent, Col. Fisher:

We had started on our way again when we got going at a little faster rate than our usual speed, say twenty miles an hour. The porter of the Pullman [coach] began to get frightened and he yelled for everybody to jump off. This sort of stampeded the passengers and several of them jumped off.[13]

Luckily, the only injury was a broken ankle.

Jumping off was not always the best idea. In 1895 the local paper in Buena Vista, Colorado, reported this somber story:

Last Friday evening, thirteen men, employed at the Alpine Tunnel, having completed their day's work, boarded an ordinary push car and started down the road to Hancock, a distance of three miles from the tunnel, where they boarded. In some manner the car got beyond their control and started down the grade at a terrific speed. The men became panic-stricken and began jumping off, thus receiving their injuries, which were not fatal except in two instances. Charles Michaelson was killed instantly.[14]

John Brady died later from head injuries received in his jump. As the paper added, however, "As far as can be ascertained, the men were alone to blame for the accident, they having started with no adequate means of checking the speed of the car."

Gilbert Lathrop described an accident that killed a young engineer:

He was switching some boxcars. During one of the moves he threw his long reverse lever into forward motion. For some unaccountable reason, the latch failed to catch. When he opened the throttle, the reverse lever smashed back and struck him in the pit of the stomach. He lived but a short time.[15]

The heavy snows of winter brought particularly difficult working conditions. On April 24, 1901, a train with two engines was fighting snowdrifts to try and reach Camp Frances, Colorado. Finally, the massive drifts stalled the train. The engineer unhooked the coaches and tried to buck the snowdrifts with just the engines. The impact of the engines on the accumulated snow, and the thundering noise of the pistons, started a snowslide that carried both of the engines off the tracks into the gulch below. Two firemen, the brakeman, and the conductor were killed.

In February 1900 a snowslide caught a train just below Crested Butte,

Colorado. Several of the cars were destroyed, but most of the train survived intact, though residents of the town were annoyed that their mail delivery was delayed by several hours.

A snowslide could be far more serious than delayed mail. On March 10, 1884, a disastrous avalanche swept through the little settlement of Wood-stock, a combination station and section house with a water tank, that was located alongside the tracks of the Denver, South Park and Pacific Railway. Thirteen of the eighteen residents, including five children, were buried under the snow. The body of Joe Royengo, the saloon keeper, was not found until the following July when a strange odor emanated from the water tank. The body was found inside it.

Railroad deaths might come from more subtle causes. Railway tunnels were sloped to provide natural ventilation to allow smoke and gas from the engines to clear out. But when a train with the firebox stoked up was parked inside a tunnel, gas and smoke could build up to fatal proportions very quickly. In June of 1895 a work crew trying to remove a cave-in inside the Alpine Tunnel on the Denver, South Park and Pacific Railway in the central mountains of Colorado was overcome by smoke and gas from a work train that had been parked in the tunnel to pump out water that had accumulated on the track. Four of the workers lost their lives. Several others were rendered unconscious by the gas but were later revived. A similar potential deathtrap existed in the snowsheds that were built over the tracks to protect trains and passengers from the severe winter weather at Corona Station on the Denver and Salt Lake Railroad. Idling trains emitted dangerous gas and smoke that could easily overcome workers and passengers.

One odd source of injuries for railroad men on the Great Plains was being shot. Apparently, cowboys on the trail could not resist shooting at the lights of passing trains, so engineers quickly learned to extinguish their head-lights and lanterns when passing near a cattle town.

Passengers were also subject to miscellaneous hazards when they traveled by railroad. A surprising number of passengers were injured by falling or jumping out of carriage windows. Of dubious comfort was the fact that railroad men were about six times more likely to suffer an accident than a passenger.

As well as being exposed to the various hazards of travel by railroad, such as train derailments and boiler explosions, passengers were at risk from contagious diseases carried by other travelers. Passenger coaches were not fumigated or sterilized, and benches and headrests received only cursory cleaning — if any. Thus, travelers with active tuberculosis or typhoid could easily leave microbes on the seats that they occupied and any surfaces that they touched for the next traveler to pick up. Uncouth passengers commonly spat on the floor, spreading disease.

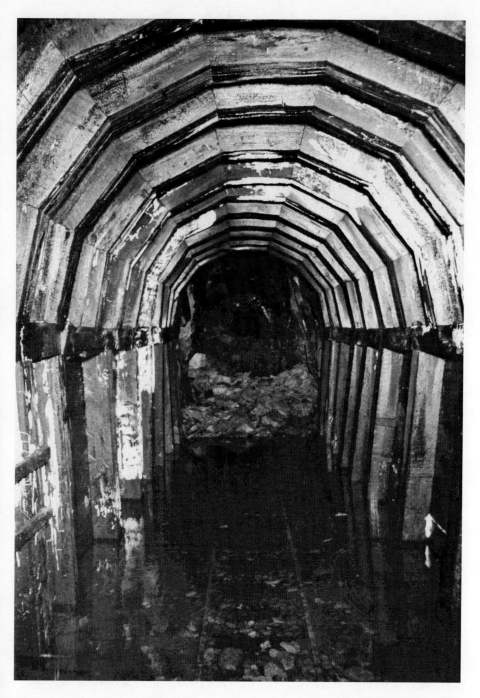

The Alpine Tunnel, which pierced the Continental Divide in central Colorado, was the scene of various railroading accidents that resulted in deaths from cave-ins or the engine gases that accumulated inside the tunnel (author's collection).

Another potential health hazard for early railroad passengers was the dubious food served at restaurants in railroad stations. Before dining cars became a standard feature on railroads, periodic train stops allowed passengers to hurriedly grab a bite to eat. The primary interest of railroad magnates was to move the maximum number of passengers in as short an amount of time as possible. As a consequence, meal stops typically lasted less than a half-hour — though some were as short as ten minutes — while the engine took on coal and water. Thus, chaos reigned when a trainload of famished passengers descended on the lunchroom of a small station. The food was often old, cold, and greasy. The coffee may have been made from nearby fragrant creek water and was often lukewarm at best. Beef was not always available, and a heavy coating of grease on meat was suspected by some passengers to be a disguise for the particular animal species that was the meat's origin.

Furthermore, it was not unknown for a train crew to be in league with the proprietor of a lunch counter to help him to maximize his revenue. One of several variations on the following basic theme might be played. Essentially, no sooner had the customers paid for their meals than the conductor would blow the "all-aboard" whistle, and the harried passengers would have to run back out to board the train again, leaving their food virtually untouched. Then the unscrupulous restaurateur would save it and bring it back out again for the next trainload of unsuspecting victims.

The man who changed this was Frederick Henry Harvey, an immigrant from London, England. After a failed attempt to open a couple of restaurants on the Kansas Pacific Railroad with an uncooperative partner, Harvey built a chain of restaurants along the Atchison, Topeka & Santa Fe railroad that served quality food at moderate prices in clean, pleasant surroundings.

For early passengers whose greasy lukewarm meals didn't agree with them, toilets on early trains emptied directly onto the track, without the use of any type of holding tank. This further created the possibility of the spread of typhoid, cholera, and similar feces-borne diseases among railroad workers and passengers, and to those who lived near the tracks.

Because accidents and injuries to engineers, firemen, brakemen, and other workers were common, most railroads retained one or more physicians on contract to treat injuries among workers and passengers. A serious accident, however, such as a train derailment or an engine boiler explosion, would require the services of as many doctors as could be mustered.

Train wrecks and accidents were certainly not unusual, as a random sampling for the Colorado Midland Railway shows. On September 18, 1887, the wreck of a construction train near Lake Ivanhoe killed three men and injured more than sixty others. On December 26, 1888, an accident twenty miles west of Leadville killed brakeman L.F. Harlan and fireman Robert Martin. On July 12, 1891, ten passengers were scalded at Aspen Junction. On July

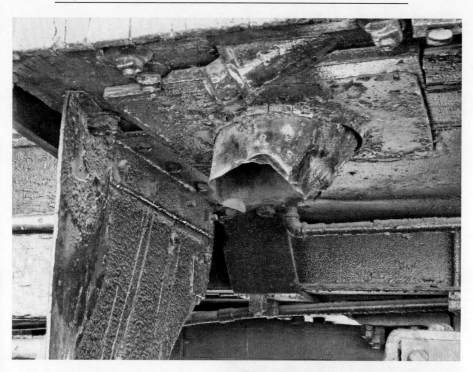

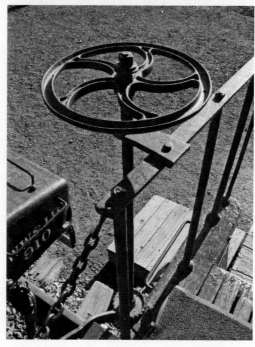

Above: Early railroad toilets had no holding tank, but simply flushed out of this vent onto the track, contributing to the spread of disease for people who lived near the railroad right-of-way. *Right:* When a train slowed or stopped, the brakemen had to run from car to car, cranking down with their hickory clubs on these wheels that set the brakes (author's collection).

15, 1891, the engineer and fireman were killed when their freight train ran away just west of Colorado Springs. A similar accident on April 30, 1892, killed the engineer. With gruesome gusto, a local newspaper reported that "both hips were crushed, his head mangled, arms broken, besides internal injuries.

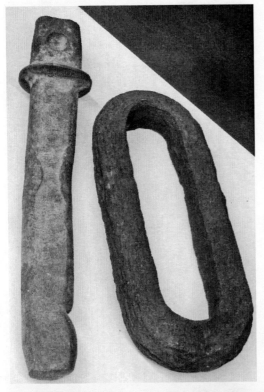

He was conscious when taken out, but died in a few hours."[16] Railroading was a very hazardous job indeed.

The second worst train wreck in the United States occurred at Eden, Colorado, just north of the town of Pueblo, on August 7, 1904. Water from a flash flood to the north roared down a creek bed under the tracks and swept away the daily express train of the Missouri Pacific as it crossed a weakened railroad bridge. The engine, coal tender, and most of the coaches plunged into the twenty-foot deep gulch below the bridge and into the raging waters. Ninety-six passengers and the operating crew, except for the fireman, were killed in the wreck. Fourteen more bodies were never found. Years later human bones were still being found in the creek bed as far away as twenty-five miles downstream.

Brakemen on railroads had particularly

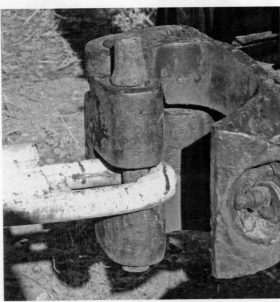

An early link-and-pin coupler for railroad cars. The oval coupler (on the top right) was placed between the two cars and secured by a pin (on the top left) on each car. This mechanism cost many a brakemen their hands and fingers. *Bottom:* This photograph shows a link-and-pin attached to half of a Janney safety coupler (author's collection).

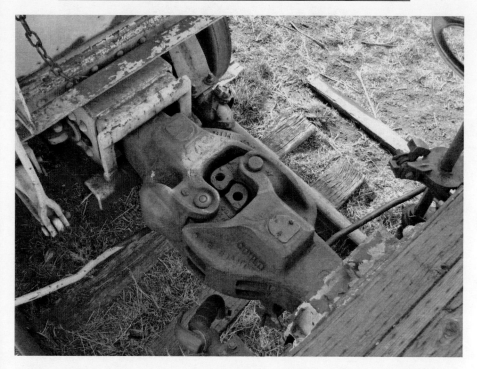

Eventually, the Janney, or "knuckle" coupler, in which the two halves of the coupler grabbed onto each other, was mandated by federal regulations for safety reasons (author's collection).

hazardous jobs. When the engines slowed down and the engineer whistled, the brakeman's task was to clamber on top of the freight cars and manually crank down on a large wheel that applied the brakes on each car. The men inserted a club — a long, stout stick made of hickory — between the spokes of the brake wheel and used the club as a handle to rapidly "club down the brakes."

Trying to retain their balance on top of a swaying freight car, perhaps at night in the dark, or with slippery snow, sleet, or ice where they were standing, and using both hands to turn the brake wheel was a daunting and dangerous task. Eventually trains were equipped with air brakes, developed by George Westinghouse, but hand brakes were the norm until well into the 1880s.

One attribute common to railroad workers was missing fingers and hands — injuries caused by the early link-and-pin couplers used to join railcars together. These couplers operated as their name implies. As the engineer backed up the train, and the cars to be joined came together, the brakeman had to place the heavy metal link on one car into a horizontal slot on the other and then drop a large metal pin into a hole on the top to attach the two cars together.

Uncoupling cars involved the reverse — trying to pull the metal pin out while the engine moved slowly to relieve the tension on the coupling. Trying to perform either of these tasks while the train was moving, perhaps made more difficult in the dark because many trains were made up at night, it was easy to get a finger or hand jammed between the heavy moving metal parts and have it crushed or severed. As Gilbert Lathrop explained, "The brakemen used pick handles to tie down hand brakes. They were a brawny lot of don't-give-a-damn young bucks. Too cocky to use the paddles provided by the company to make couplings with links and pins, most of them had from one to four fingers missing off their right or left hands."[17] In 1873, Eli Janney patented a safety coupler — called the "knuckle" coupler — that was controlled by a lever outside the car to join railroad cars together automatically. This device did not come into general use until 1893, when the old link-and-pin couplers were outlawed by the Railway Appliance and Safety Act.

CHAPTER TEN

Patent Medicines

An important part of the story of medicine in the Old West in the late 1800s and early 1900s was the use of patent medicines. The scarcity of doctors in the Old West, and the high cost of medical care, helped create an enormous popularity for self-medication with these questionable medicines.

Patent medicines, also sometimes called "proprietary medicines," were a series of pills, tonics, and potions, concocted by various manufacturers, that were based on their own ideas of healing and were mostly without any curative powers. Patent medicines were not regulated and were freely available from any drugstore, from a medicine show salesman, or directly through the mail from the manufacturer. The use of patent medicines started to flourish in the 1870s and peaked in the 1880s, but their popularity continued until about the 1930s. Some of these medicines are still sold in modified form today. Hinkley's Bone Liniment, first made in 1856, was still being manufactured and sold in 1959.

The Federal Food, Drug and Cosmetic Act was passed in 1906 to regulate food and drugs and ensure that they were manufactured to appropriate standards of purity. The Act also required that labels of drugs containing narcotics, such as opium or morphine, indicate the amount and strength of these substances. The Harrison Narcotic Act, passed in 1914, regulated the manufacture, importation, sale, and use of opium, cocaine, and other narcotics. There were exceptions in the federal law for small amounts of these drugs, but some states overruled the exemptions and maintained tight restrictions on all narcotics. Before the passage of these laws, manufacturers of patent medicines were essentially free to promote and sell whatever they wanted.

The use of patent medicines grew out of the practice of using family folk remedies. Given a lack of trust in doctors and their ability to cure disease in the late 1800s, manufacturers of patent medicines advertised their wares with clever marketing psychology. Unscrupulous manufacturers produced medicines that they felt would cater to the craving of the uneducated masses for a simple, cheap, effective cure that they could administer themselves. Advertising was

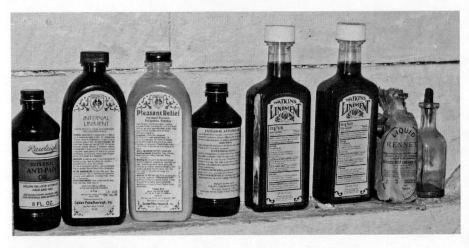

Patent medicines like these — intended to treat almost any ailment — line a shelf in a pioneer cabin (author's collection).

often aimed at the pioneer wife on the frontier, who was usually the one who administered medical care for her family. Manufacturers created a product and then generated sales and a demand for it by intense advertising campaigns.

Manufacturers spent hundreds of thousands of dollars in advertising to convince the masses that they had to rush out and buy the product or immediately send away for it in the mail. Part of the psychology of the patent medicine manufacturers was that most of the readers of their advertising enjoyed reading vivid and morbid descriptions of illnesses.[1] If the advertising copy was cleverly worded, many of these readers would agree that they probably had some of these same symptoms. Luckily for the consumer, many diseases were self-limiting and eventually cured themselves, given sufficient time. However, the use of a patent medicine often gave the appearance of curing a particular disease or diseases.

Patent medicines were claimed to offer cures for a long list of illnesses, including such diverse ailments as jaundice, dropsy, yellow fever, biliousness, tiredness, vertigo, flatulence, heartburn, kidney and liver diseases, cramps, vomiting, stomach distress, acid digestion, bloating, coughs, consumption, epilepsy, migraine, low blood pressure, high blood pressure, gallstones, strokes, bronchitis, whooping cough, and tuberculosis. In other words, almost everything. Cures for coughs, asthma, and consumption were popular in advertising because these diseases were so widespread.

Parker's Ginger Tonic claimed to cure "disease arising from defective nutrition, impure blood, and exhaustion." It was also touted for asthma, indigestion, skin eruptions, kidney disorders, malaria, and female complaints. Hagar's Chill and Fever Specific offered basically the same cures. J.O. Aldrich's

Lung Salve was recommended for lung troubles, croup, and sore throats, as well as burns, bruises, and dog bites. Among its more questionable claims was that it was good for peritonitis, appendicitis, and inflammation of the liver and kidneys.

In the late 1800s the time was right for patent medicines. Their use provided an alternative to the conventional medicine of the day. Instead of putting up with medical treatment that consisted primarily of the unpleasant routines of bleeding or purging, or the risks of gruesome surgery and subsequent infection, it was easier to take a few swigs of a proprietary medicine that promised to cure almost every ailment. If the patient did not have some serious or life-threatening disease, these remedies may have actually been safer than conventional treatments. To many people, dosing one's self or family with a patent medicine that promised a guaranteed cure for almost everything seemed as reasonable as undergoing some of the less attractive conventional treatments that were available.

The name "patent medicine" originated in Europe. In England, royal patents were granted for proprietary concoctions, hence the name "patent medicine" was used to describe them. American patent medicines were not "patented" in the same sense that inventions were registered and patented with the U.S. Patent Office. Instead they were proprietary drugs with secret formulas. If American "patent" medicines had been patented through the Patent Office in the same way as inventions, a manufacturer would have been required to disclose the formula and it would become common knowledge for competing manufacturers. Indeed, it would have been difficult to patent these medicines in the ordinary sense because their formulas were frequently changed by the manufacturers as they saw fit.

The bottles used for these medicines, however, typically had unique shapes, colors, and labels to distinguish them from their competition. So instead of patenting the medicine itself, the labels and designs of the containers were copyrighted in order to protect brand recognition.

The "medicines" inside the bottles were not regulated before the passage of the Pure Food and Drug Act of 1906. Ingredients did not have to be proven safe or effective, and there were no regulations for the claims of effectiveness on the ailments that the medicine was supposed to cure, as there are today. For example, an 1870 advertisement for Katalysine Water grandly claimed that it could cure gout, rheumatism, diabetes, neuralgia, dropsy, hemorrhoids, asthma, catarrh, diseases of the skin, and nervous prostration. Quite an array of ailments to be cured by a glass of mineral water.

Claims were boundless. Dr. Simmons proclaimed, "The cowboys carry Simmons Liver Regulator with them and take it when they feel bilious." He claimed that even Wyatt Earp and Doc Holliday had been saved from bilious attacks by his wonderful medicine.

Patent medicines were often simply potions heavily laced with opium or alcohol which were intended to make the user feel good. Others were outright frauds, such as Vital Sparks, a medicine touted to boost male virility, that consisted of pieces of hard black candy rolled in powdered aloes. The label on the small pasteboard package said that it was "God's Great Gift to MEN," the inference being obvious.

In time, patent medicines became identified with "snake oil" and "snake oil salesmen." This came about because oil made from snakes was supposed to be a particularly valuable remedy. One folk remedy, for example, was to use scorpion oil as a diuretic in cases of venereal disease. Rattlesnake oil was prized above all others. However, in spite of advertising, even snake oil was not always what it claimed to be. One popular "snake oil" was actually wintergreen oil dissolved in white gasoline.

Patent medicine salesmen also became identified with the name "charlatan." The original meaning of this word did not have the bad connotation it later received. It started innocently enough with the Italian word *ciarlatano*, which meant "to sell drugs in public places." It later came to be associated with an untrustworthy impostor who pretended to have knowledge that he did not, because so many patent medicines proved ineffective.

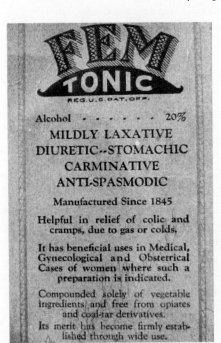

One of many patent medicines. The label speaks for itself (author's collection).

The Medicines

Alcohol, opium, and cocaine were common ingredients in patent medicines. Both Kendall's Balsam and Old Sachem Bitters contained opium and alcohol. Wyeth's New Enteritis Pills and Mrs. Winslow's Soothing Syrup contained morphine. As might be imagined, the effects of these drugs made them popular among users. To offset any concerns among the consuming public, manufacturers claimed with great aplomb that such ingredients were "not harmful," "non-addictive," and "natural remedies," when drinking potions that contained opium and cocaine were anything but harmless and non-addictive. Jaynes Carminative, for example, contained 23 percent alcohol and about a grain of opium in a fluid ounce. The normal recommended dose of laudanum to treat dysentery was six milligrams.[2] One grain was equivalent to sixty milligrams of opium, so Jayne's Carminative contained ten times the usual medically-recommended dose.

Dr. King's New Discovery for Consumption, claiming itself to be "the only sure cure for consumption in the world," contained morphine and chloroform. The chloroform stopped the coughing, and the morphine put the user into a drug-induced haze. In the meantime, the tuberculosis raged unchecked, and the victim felt no need for further treatment as he was not coughing and felt relatively good. Dr. J.C. Fahey's Pepsin Anodyne claimed to be "absolutely harmless," and it "contains no laudanum." That was true; however, in the fine print, the carton admitted that it contained chloral hydrate and morphine. A fine distinction indeed.

"Herbal," "vegetable," or "natural" ingredients were often part of the claims, as the medicines included substances such as aloe, mandrake, colocynth, digitalis, fish oil, and sassafras. Many of the ingredients were laxative or diuretic in nature, so that the user felt like the medicine was doing something. Other, more potent ingredients that were used included creosote, turpentine, kerosene, arsenic, prussic acid (cyanide), and strychnine. Some patent medicines contained ingredients that tasted awful to appeal to those consumers who thought that disease could only be driven from the body by a cure that tasted disgusting.

Addiction to patent medicine was common because narcotic drugs, such as opium, cocaine, and morphine, were not controlled substances at the time. There were no legal limits on prescribing opium in various forms, and a large percentage of women were addicted to drugs as a result of frequent use of opium-based patent medicines, many of which were promoted specifically for "the diseases of women" (or some such similar wording).

Patent medicines also commonly contained a high percentage of alcohol. Twenty-five percent of Burdock Blood Bitters was alcohol. Hinkley's Bone Liniment contained 47 percent alcohol, much reduced from its original 1856 version of 86 percent alcohol by volume.

Other examples were Baker's Stomach Bitters and Limerick's Liniment, which also claimed to be good for diseases in horses. Livestock was apparently the recipient of several of these strange alcoholic brews. Dr. A.W. Allen's Southern Liniment claimed to be good for rheumatism, neuralgia, sprains, burns, bruises, and colic. To appeal to rural customers, it also claimed to be "the only certain remedy for blind staggers in horses."

In 1878 the Internal Revenue Service, noting that Hostetter's Celebrated Stomach Bitters was being sold in saloons in Sitka, Alaska, as an alcoholic beverage, were of the decided opinion that the drink should be taxed as liquor. Hostetter's Bitters, promoted as being good for the treatment of dyspepsia,

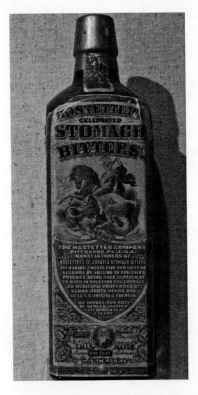

ague, dysentery, colic, and nervous prostration, contained between 44 and 47 percent alcohol before it was later reduced by the Pure Food and Drug Act to 25 percent. In 1920, pressure from the American Medical Association over Hostetter's claims caused the company to change the name from Hostetter's Celebrated Stomach Bitters to Hostetter's Celebrated Stomachic Bitters—another fine, but meaningless, distinction. A "stomachic" is defined as: "...given to improve the tone of the stomach and to increase the appetite by stimulating the secretion of gastric juice."[3]

These alcohol solutions were essentially tinctures, or drugs dissolved in alcohol. One contemporary medical advice book even said, "Though a convenient form of preserving some medicines ... the use of them frequently induces habits of intemperance."[4]

Many patent medicines proclaimed themselves to be a "female remedy"; thus, women who swore that a drop of liquor would never pass their lips could happily take a spoonful or two a day of an alcohol-laced patent medicine and still believe that they never touched strong drink. A clue to the contents of many of these "medicines," however, should have been obvious, because the name "bitters" was used as a generic term for medicinal alcohol with herbs dissolved in it. Other tonics that were high in alcohol were Faith Whitcomb's Nerve Bitters (20 percent), Burdoch Blood Bitters (25 percent), Flint's Quaker Bitters (23 percent), the hypocritically-named Luther's Temperance Bitters (17 percent), and Dr. Walker's Temperance Bitters.

Peruna, one of the most prominent patent remedies in the country, contained 28 percent alcohol. The

Hostetter's Celebrated Stomach Bitters was one of the most popular of the patent medicines—and one of the highest in alcoholic content (author's collection).

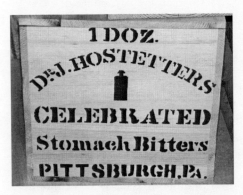

It was so popular that it was literally sold by the case (author's collection).

Peruna prescription was to drink three wine glasses of the medicine in a forty-five minute period, a remedy that should have caused even the most dyspeptic individuals to feel quite mellow. By comparison, most wines today contain 12 percent alcohol.

The high alcohol content in a patent medicine was the source of an ironic turn (tinged with black humor) when Perry Davis, the manufacturer of Dr. Davis' Celebrated Pain Killer, was preparing a new batch of "medicine" on March 25, 1844. As he worked, the alcohol that was the main ingredient caught fire and badly burned his face and hands.

From their beginnings, patent medicines often retained the nineteenth century focus of frontier medicine on the bowels. One early remedy, named *Aqua anti torminales*, was touted as a cure for "the Griping of the Guts, and the Wind Cholick; but preventeth that woeful Distemper of the Dry Belly Ach."[5]

Many patent medicines were laxatives or purgatives in disguise, consisting of such old standbys as aloes, jalap, rhubarb, colocynth, and senna, just the same as conventional medicines of the time. Because these ingredients were based on plant extracts, the medicines were promoted as "natural," "Nature's remedy," "pure vegetable remedy," and other similar soothing, glowing terms. Proprietary medicines equated purgatives with purifying the blood — the old humoral theory reincarnated — thus, many patent medicines trumpeted that they would remove impurities from the blood. In reality, their primary effect was to remove the contents of the bowels.

One such patent medicine was Brandreth's Vegetable Universal Pills. Benjamin Brandreth's advertising, still focusing on the idea of purging from ancient heroic medicine, claimed that impurities of the blood were the cause of all diseases. Even as late as the 1880s, company advertising claimed that people who were ill carried "corrupt humors" in their bowels and blood, but that these could be "expelled" — so to speak — by sufficient use of the company's pills. The medicine contained in Brandreth's Vegetable Universal Pills was compounded from aloes, colocynth, and gamboge. This was indeed a combination that was guaranteed to expel everything. One customer proudly claimed that her husband fed the pills as a preventative to his horses, oxen, cats, dogs, and pigs, with the same wonderful results.

Regular and energetic purging was considered necessary by patent medicine manufacturers to keep the customer's system "flowing" correctly. One ardent manufacturer of patent medicines, James Morison, believed that the stomach and bowels could not be purged too much. His belief was that the single cause for all disease was "bad blood." His solution was frequent use of his Vegetable Universal Pills.

The primary ingredients in Paine's Celery Compound were celery and coca — and an unhealthy 21 percent dose of alcohol. Its popularity lasted into the 1920s. Manufactured by the Wells & Richardson Company of Burlington, Vermont, it was described by them as a nerve tonic — and presumably the coca and alcohol did indeed quiet the disposition. Its advertising claimed, "It drives out poisonous humors of the blood, purifying and enriching it and so overcoming those diseases resulting from impure or impoverished blood."[6] It also functioned as a laxative, claiming by this action to strengthen the stomach and aid the digestion. Other claims were that it acted as a diuretic to cure kidney and urinary disorders, and was good for biliousness, jaundice, constipation, piles (hemorrhoids), rheumatism, neuralgia, and female complaints.

Dr. J.B. Kendall's Quick Relief, manufactured in Enosburg Falls, Vermont, was described as being for both external and internal use. Taken externally, it was for rheumatism, neuralgia, toothache, and sprains. Taken internally, it was recommended for cramps or curing pain in the bowels or stomach. The label claimed that it contained 73 percent alcohol. Remarkable indeed, as most gins, vodkas, and whiskies today contain about 40 percent alcohol. As its name implied, the alcohol level in Kendall's medicine should have provided quick relief and forgetfulness for many ailments.

The label for Warner's Safe Cure promoted a nautical theme and called itself "the beacon light of safety to all wrecked by disease." It was described as an "unfailing specific" for kidney, liver, bladder, blood, and female disorders. Stafford's Olive Tar was guaranteed to be a specific treatment for all types of tuberculosis, whether it was taken internally, applied externally, or the vapor was inhaled. Another patent medicine that was claimed to be a sure cure for consumption was Hale's Honey of Hoarhound and Tar.

J.S. Merrell's FEM tonic contained 20 percent alcohol. It claimed to be mildly laxative, diuretic-stomachic, carminative, and antispasmodic. In spite of this, the manufacturer's claims weren't as exaggerated as most patent medicines. However, users were left to draw their own conclusions as to its efficacy, because the label said, "It has beneficial uses in Medicinal, Gynecological and Obstetrical Cases of women where such a preparation is indicated." A veritable masterpiece of vague wording.

The J.A. Slocum Company, manufacturing chemists of New York, claimed on the label of its product Psychine (containing only 10 percent alcohol) that it "Improves the Tone and Vigor of the Stomach and Bowels and thus increases the Powers of Digestion." Again, an emphasis on the bowels. The manufacturer apparently wanted the user to go through a bottle quickly, because the directions for use were to take a tablespoonful before and after each meal, and upon retiring. Users of the tonic must have felt quite mellow and lighter in their wallets at the same time, as the cost was three dollars a bottle — a hefty price in an age when that was the average daily wage of a gold miner.

One of the most famous patent medicines was Lydia Pinkham's Vegetable Compound, which was advertised as the "only positive cure and legitimate remedy for the peculiar weaknesses and ailments of women." It was developed by housewife Mrs. Lydia Pinkham of Lynn, Massachusetts, who started selling her home herbal remedy in 1873. In 1875 her tonic sold for a dollar a bottle. She claimed that it contained purely vegetable ingredients, derived from various roots. This tonic at one time contained 21 percent alcohol, which was used, so the company claimed, "as a solvent and preservative." Another ingredient was a large proportion of opium. Pinkham's Vegetable Compound was specifically recommended for pneumonia, kidney disease, constipation, tuberculosis, appendicitis, "the recurrent problems of women," and "female complaints and weaknesses." It even claimed to cure infertility.

In a stroke of marketing genius, the Pinkham family put Lydia's picture on the label, making her the most recognized woman in America at that time. Her grandmotherly look and kindly smile appealed to readers of Pinkham's advertising and users of the medicine, and gave them confidence in its curative abilities. Shrewd

Lydia Pinkham's kindly face on bottles of her patent medicine made her one of the most recognized women in America at the time (author's collection).

marketing using this promotion resulted in a huge volume of sales, and by 1881, the Pinkham Company was grossing $30,000 a month. Other clever marketing techniques were heavy advertising in newspapers and a personal reply from Mrs. Pinkham to those who wrote to her for advice. Her advice continued, supplied by a team of company writers, until the early 1900s, even after she died in 1883. The company published a popular booklet called *Guide for Women* that was aimed specifically at female users and described the benefits of the medicine for them. It contained a quite frank discussion, for the times, of female physiology and the disorders that women were subject to. When first published, the guide had four pages. It turned out to be immensely popular and by 1901 had grown to sixty-two pages.

Indian Cures

Another popular theme among patent medicines was American Indian remedies. To the public, this implied secret Indian cures that had been handed down from generation to generation by those who were assumed to be Indian healers and medicine men. They were marketed as secret bottled tonics, the formulas of which were supposedly entrusted to the manufacturer by Indian medicine men seeking to better mankind. Typically they were compounded from herbs, roots, and bark, properly "soaked in alcohol," which gave the user a pleasant euphoric after-effect when the medicine was used.

A clever design for the label of some of the Indian patent medicines was to add a drawing of an American Indian in full headdress. This was to manipulate the customer into thinking that the contents were an age-old natural remedy.

A typical "Indian" patent medicine was *Re-Cu-Ma*, which proudly called itself "the great Indian root and herb tonic." It was supposed to be particularly good for the blood, liver, kidneys, and stomach, and it was promoted as a remedy for rheumatism, constipation, indigestion, malaise, and biliousness. The recommended dose was one tablespoon taken three times a day.

Indian themes were also promoted by the Oregon Indian Medicine Company, which was organized and promoted by Donald McKay from Oregon. His cure-all (at 20 percent alcohol) went under a similar Indian-sounding name of *Ka-Ton-Ka*. It was supposedly prepared deep in the forests of Oregon by the Modoc and the Nez Percé Indians of the Northwest, but in reality it was made by a drug manufacturer in Corry, Pennsylvania. Federal chemists who analyzed the Great Indian Medicine as part of a fraudulent advertising investigation declared that the ingredients were alcohol, sugar, aloes, and baking soda. One of the company's best sellers was Donald McKay's Indian Worm Eradicator. Others were Nez Percé Catarrh Snuff and Modoc Oil.

The most successful of the Indian patent medicines were the series of Kickapoo Indian Medicines. The company was founded by John E. Healy and Charles (Texas Charlie) H. Bigelow. Healy's previous experience included selling liver pads for aches and pains, and a medicine named the "King of Pain."

The Kickapoo company was based in Connecticut but was shrewdly named after the Kickapoo Indian Nation in Oklahoma. The company's staple medicine was Kickapoo Indian Sagwa, which was claimed to cure dyspepsia, rheumatism, and diseases of the kidneys and liver. Its primary effect, however, was to act as a laxative. Ingredients in Sagwa included herbs, roots, bark, and buffalo fat. And, of course, the medicine included a healthy dose of alcohol. Other nostrums for the company were Kickapoo Indian Oil, a mystical cure for multiple ills, which also claimed to cure nervous and inflammatory diseases. The medicine may have helped some nervous people, as it contained enough alcohol to be a relaxant and a marginal pain killer. Kickapoo Indian Salve was available to cure skin diseases, and Kickapoo Indian Worm Killer was promoted for ridding the user of seatworms and pinworms. Kickapoo Indian Prairie Plant was available for those with "female complaints."

The Kickapoo company was a master at advertising. Their campaigns included pamphlets, magazines that contained Indian-related adventure stories and poems, company souvenirs, and a host of supplemental literature, all of which was oriented towards selling their brand of patent medicines. They promoted shows that featured performers in Indian costumes, with frequent breaks in the show to sell their patent medicines. They even built an Indian village behind the company headquarters in New Haven.

Other popular medicines were those with an oriental theme. Most people associated the Far East with ancient wisdom, mysterious cures, and secret remedies.

Advertising

The market for patent medicines was fanned to fever pitch by advertising campaigns. In the 1880s and 1890s a glut of advertising that appeared everywhere was used to try to get people to forsake the old family remedies and use patent medicines instead. The overwhelming claims and cures were limited only by the copy writers' imagination. At one point in his career, even the famous showman P.T. Barnum wrote advertising copy for a cure for baldness.

Manufacturers coined vague descriptions for use in their advertising. Imaginary ailments, such as "catarrh of the liver," "turbid biliousness," "acid fermentation," and "atonic dyspepsia" were not unusual.

The producers of patent medicines pioneered methods of advertising that exaggerated the benefits of the product, and psychologically manipulated and deceived the reader, both at the same time. In this manner the manufacturers created tremendously profitable businesses. Most bottles of tonic sold for between one and five dollars. Most cost anywhere from fifteen to twenty-five cents to manufacture. The medicines were compounded in large quantities. The factory for Walker's California Vinegar Bitter had a manufacturing capacity of 44,000 gallons.

Consumers were bombarded with claims of better health by seductive advertisements in newspapers and magazines, on billboards, in brochures, and on posters, all of which trumpeted the benefits of the manufacturer's particular nostrum. Several factors helped create the subsequent boom in the patent medicine business. Expansion of the railroad system into small towns brought more salesmen and medicine shows; expansion of the postal system made ordering easier and sped delivery of the medicine directly to the home; and an explosion in the number of newspapers in small towns across the country allowed advertising to constantly cajole the consumer into buying the product. In the early days, calendars were difficult to get. As a result, manufacturers of patent medicines found that providing calendars that touted their products was a good advertising ploy.

Popular magazines of the time, such as *Harper's Magazine, Collier's*, and *Atlantic Monthly*, carried full-page advertisements for patent medicines. Estimates are that by the 1870s, fully one-fourth of all print advertising was for patent medicines.

Not everyone was convinced by this overwhelming mass of advertising. One drugstore in Topeka, Kansas, displayed a sign that read: "We sell patent medicines, but we do not recommend them."[7]

Heavy advertising of patent medicines and "secret remedies" attracted the attention of the orthodox medical establishment, and there was a running battle between the regular doctors and the purveyors of patent medicines. Doctors tried to warn potential users of the dangers of self-medication and blindly treating the wrong disease. In rebuttal, the manufacturers of patent medicines said that the medical establishment was trying to suppress medical breakthroughs and treatments for diseases that the doctors could not cure. When physicians protested many of the exaggerated and optimistic claims, they were seen as being an organized opposition to "the competition."

Medicine Shows

A popular technique used to promote the sales of patent medicines was the medicine show, a combination of carnival, side show, and sales pitch, which became a popular form of entertainment during the late nineteenth century. Combining elements of circus performances, Wild West shows, vaudeville troupes, and minstrel musicals, these traveling entertainment shows were intended to attract an audience and then sell them patent medicines. Medicine shows were presented all across the United States and even around the world.[8]

A similar formula for patent medicine shows had originated in Europe. Actors entertained with skits or a short play, either a drama or with comedy elements, and performers sang, danced, or performed circus-type acts. These turns at entertainment were intermingled with a pitch from the salesman. This resulted in patent medicines being sold in a carnival-like atmosphere, with snake oil salesmen selling from the back of a wagon on street corners. The sales pitch was delivered with a rapid patter that was a combination vaudeville act and circus come-on. Salesmen promised that their product would provide a sure-fire cure that would take care of all ailments. People were drawn to the free entertainment and even enjoyed listening to the salesman's pitch.

Indians might be hired to perform dances or native songs to add to the atmosphere for Indian remedies. The Kickapoo company's traveling show was made up to look like an Indian village, complete with scouts and Indian braves to add a colorful flavor to the medicine pitch. In the late 1880s, the company had several dozen shows on the road at the same time, some performing the same show in Europe and as far away as Australia.

The first medicine shows were fairly small and featured a pitchman backed by a few entertainers, such as singers, musicians, jugglers, or acrobats. The shows traveled from town to town, often appearing in mining camps and small frontier towns, setting up a temporary stage for entertainment and sales. The pitchman was usually a distinguished-looking older man dressed in a frock coat and top hat (like a country doctor) to add credibility to the sales pitch. His imposing appearance was good for selling to naïve and gullible audiences. In some cases the salesman conferred the title of "Doctor" on himself to add to his credentials for recommending and selling the product.

Medicine shows grew in popularity from about 1870 to 1920, providing entertainment for the masses when the troupe hit town. During the latter part of the nineteenth century, the larger traveling medicine shows, featuring professional entertainers who sang, danced, performed magic acts, or exhibitions of trick shooting, were standard fare for entertainment in small towns. After the show the audience was encouraged to buy the sponsor's "tonics" and "elixirs."

The members of the medicine show entertainment acts doubled as salespeople at this point, and the troupe sold as much as they could, moving among the gathered crowd and showing the wares. Shills—the confederates of the pitchman—started the sales rolling by eagerly buying the first bottles or boxes when the pitchmen held them up. Other shills in the crowd might yell out that they had been "cured" of some dread disease by this particular remedy. After that, sales came fast and furious. Other subtle inducements to buy might be added. Kickapoo Indian Worm Killer reportedly sold well (for twenty-five cents a box) after the audience at their medicine shows saw huge tapeworms (purchased from local stockyards before the show) prominently displayed next to advertisements for the remedy. .

Then everyone left town quietly and quickly in case angry customers returned for a refund, or even revenge, if the "cure" didn't live up to its advertised claims.

The Peculiar Role of Women's Corsets

As part of their advertising, manufacturers of patent medicines promoted and capitalized on a series of symptoms that they termed "diseases of women," "diseases peculiar to women," or some other vague verbiage. The interpretation of what this actually meant was left to the reader. Many have assumed these ailments to be due to female biology, such as menstrual cramps,

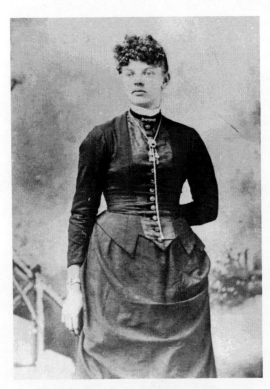

The Victorian ideal of beauty was a full figure, ideally weighing 160 or 170 pounds when the typical height for a woman was about 5'3" or 5'4" tall (Glenn Kinnaman, Colorado and Western History Collection).

pregnancy issues, and mental aberrations, such as the popular Victorian disease of "hysteria" that was attributed to women's psychological makeup. Other evidence, however, showed that there was also an additional, lesser-known, legitimate physical basis for some of these "female complaints."

The second half of the nineteenth century saw a rise in the use of tight corsets for women, and the manufacture of corsets became a thriving industry. The Victorian era was the age when the ideal of femininity was a wasp-shaped figure with tiny waist, a large bosom, and hefty hips. Men were supposed to be able to span a woman's waist with their two hands. A twenty or twenty-one inch waist was considered to be perfect. One prevalent idea was that an appropriate waist size for women should be the same as their age when they married.

Though wearing corsets has been popularly attributed to upper-class Victorian women, fashion historians have shown that working-class women considered corsets an essential part of their daily dress, if for no other reason than they wanted to emulate their employers and social betters.

A by-product of the tightly-laced corsets used to achieve this hour glass-shaped figure was that the garment placed tremendous downward pressure on the abdomen and pelvic organs. Contemporary medical writings showed that there was a relationship between constricting corsets and "female complaints."

The same pressure was exerted upwards on the lungs, stomach, and heart. Not surprisingly, women who wore tight corsets commented on a choking sensation and inability to breathe properly. A few enlightened physicians confirmed that pressure on the abdomen from wearing tight

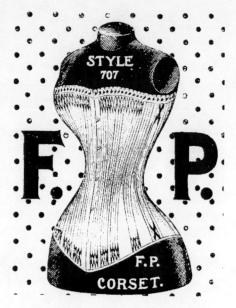

The tight corset worn by a Victorian woman produced her hourglass figure, but caused internal problems due to downward pressure on pelvic organs and upward pressure on the heart and lungs (Glenn Kinnaman, Colorado and Western History Collection).

corsets resulted in a variety of physical illnesses, ranging from nausea, a lack of appetite, headaches, constipation, disrupted menstrual cycles, fainting due to difficulty breathing, and the most serious—uterine displacement. Pressure on the liver, stomach, small intestines, and large intestine created a sense of uneasiness, a sense of pelvic weight, back pain, and aching of the inner thighs. Other symptoms included a pale complexion, palpitations, loss of breath upon exertion, swollen legs at the end of the day, and "bilious attacks." These problems did not appear in men or thin women, and were relieved — not surprisingly — by bed rest, when the corset was not worn.

An advertisement for Lydia Pinkham's tonic quoted one woman as saying that she had symptoms that included a weak stomach, indigestion, the feeling of bearing down (as for a bowel movement) all the time, and pains in the groin and thighs. The advertisement went on to say, "An unhealthy condition of the female organs can produce all the above symptoms in the same person."[9] The recommended cure for resolution of these symptoms was, of course, to take a regular course of Pinkham's patent medicine.

There was even an injury that was referred to as "chicken breast," in which the extreme pressure of some tightly-laced corsets pushed the lower ribs inward so far that they rode up over the sternum (breast bone) and fractured. The lower (or vertebral) ribs, the so-called "floating ribs," which do not attach to the breast bone, were most at risk for this injury. To prevent this, and enhance their tiny waists, some women actually had the lowest ribs on each side surgically removed in their quest for what they perceived to be "the perfect figure."

The delicate Victorian phrase "diseases peculiar to women" generally referred to uterine displacement, a condition that was accompanied by severe abdominal pain. Evidence for the extent of this problem can be seen by the invention and availability in the Victorian era of a large number of pessaries— mechanical devices that were inserted into the vagina to hold the uterus in place after it became displaced. Doctors seeking the female trade advertised that they supplied a wide range of "supporting devices."

Promoting what would appear to be contradictory goals, several proprietary designs of corset were available with a built-in pessary — so that the corset was tightly-laced and pushed the uterus downwards, while the pessary attempted to push it back up again. Use of these devices could lead to further "female problems" due to infection or damage to internal organs.

Uterine displacement occurred in Victorian times just as frequently in unmarried women as in married women with children, thus indicating that previous childbirth was not the cause. The condition often went untreated because most women were reluctant to confide in a male doctor and undergo a highly intimate and embarrassing physical examination.[10] Pain was often relieved at night when the corset was removed, but many physicians did not make the connection.

Self-treatment to relieve the pain and discomfort was to use morphine, opium, laudanum, or a patent medicine that included these ingredients to dull the pain. The undesired side effect, of course, was eventual drug addiction.

Medical Quackery

Dubious medical care was not restricted to patent medicines. The discovery and legitimate uses for electricity, radioactivity, and magnetism were quickly followed by their incorporation into a host of medical devices, many of which had no legitimate basis. Part of this was due to the aura of new discoveries and their use in medicine, and partly it was because these devices appeared to "do" something by creating burning or tingling sensations in the skin.

By the 1870s, electric "treatments" were becoming common. Two sources were used for the electricity. One was galvanic currents, or direct current, from a battery. The other was faradic current, similar to the alternating current (AC) supplied to the wall sockets in today's home electric power.[11] Galvanic currents were used to stimulate localized muscle contractions (for example, to stimulate the bowels). Again there was the old obsession with the bowels, only now the idea of bowel consciousness and purgation was reincarnated by means of an electric current. Faradic currents were used to give the body a more powerful stimulus, and was often used, in the familiar fashion of the day, to stimulate the bowels.

Some of the legitimate medical uses of electrotherapy were to relieve pain and headaches, to cauterize wounds, and to stimulate paralyzed muscles.[12] Confusion was generated in consumers because legitimate medical doctors endorsed electrotherapy for legitimate medical uses. It was an easy step for the charlatans to step in and offer electric cures for anything and everything. Popular devices were electric "invigorators," electric belts, vibration devices, and magnetic collars. These devices were promoted to "energize" the body by replacing lost energy and creating new energy.

The failure to produce an effective cure after pretentious claims for various electric machines led to these devices being categorized as "quack" medical devices. Quack is an abbreviation for "quacksalver," a sixteenth-century name given to a person who sold salves with a fast sales pitch, or patter, that sounded like a duck quacking. The shortened name became applied to a fraudulent promoter of bogus "medical" devices or to the device itself.

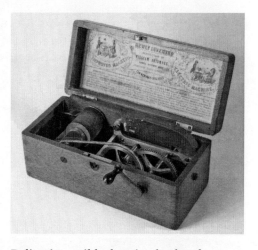

By the 1880s, quack medical practitioners had expanded the use of electrotherapy to treat a wide variety of ailments, from poor eyesight to sexual problems, none of which were curable by electricity. Various electrodes were available for insertion into the natural body openings (such as nose, ears, vagina, and anus) to provide specialized "treatments."[13]

A common method of the application of electricity was to give the patient a mild electrical shock — enough to produce a tingling sensation. Typical of these

Delivering mild electric shocks, from devices such as this hand-cranked generator manufactured by William Skidmore, was a popular technique among the manufacturers of quack medical devices to make the user feel like the device actually did something (author's collection).

devices was Davis & Kidder's Patent Magneto Electric Machine. Produced in the 1880s, this machine was advertised as a cure for "nervous diseases." The user applied two electrodes to the desired part of the body, then cranked the handle of a generator to deliver electric current.

Moorhead's Graduated Magnetic Machine, first manufactured in 1847, contained two metallic handles that were held by users, while the machine sent current through their hands. Moorhead claimed that disease was the result of "imperfect vital forces." His machine was supposed to cure ills by recharging the body with electricity. When users felt the definite tingle generated in the hands and wrists, they became believers.

A period starting in about 1880, and lasting until about 1920, was the golden age of quack electric therapy, and both legitimate physicians and quack medicine men came up with increasingly widespread "cures." Much of this development paralleled the rise in electrification of American cities and homes, confirming the belief in consumers that electricity could be effectively used to cure a myriad of ailments. Starting in about 1890, physicians realized the problem that had been unleashed by the use of bogus electric devices, and they started to campaign against these quack devices and their promoters.

One of the more peculiar, but very popular, electric treatments was the use of electric belts, the first of which appeared on the market as early as the 1870s. One of the best-known was J.L. Pulvermacher's belt, first marketed in 1875 by the Pulvermacher Galvanic Company. The belts were made from cloth interwoven with metallic wires on the inside that contacted the skin and produced a tingling sensation as current was passed through what were effectively multiple electrodes surrounding the waist.

Other examples were belts made by the German Electric Company of New York and Addison's Electric Belt, both of which were heavily promoted by marketers and often sold by direct advertising in newspapers and magazines, and door-to-door by aggressive salesmen. Like the patent medicines, outlandish claims were made for the efficacy of these belts, promising a wide range of cures and catering to the general public's fear of disease. Like the electrotherapy machines, electric belts claimed to restore lost energy and health though the application of electrical force.

An optional accessory to Pulvermacher's electric belts was a "suspensory appliance" attached to the belt. This was a wire mesh and cloth bag that surrounded the male genitals and exposed them to a mild galvanic current. Its avowed purpose was to restore "lost vigor." The loss of "vigor" and "vitality," along with similar terms, were Victorian euphemisms for sexual dysfunction, such as impotence and erectile disorders. Advertising for cures typically showed idealized drawings of muscular naked male figures wearing the belt and suspensory. The objective was to create the impression in the reader that he too could increase erectile performance and sexual prowess by purchasing and wearing an electric belt.

Electric belts were popularly sold by mail order houses because, in this way, they could be privately purchased and delivered to the buyer's home with the utmost discretion for a problem that most men would not want to share with the family physician. Belt manufacturers trumpeted and emphasized the problems and symptoms of sexual inadequacy so that they could induce the fear of sexual failure in potential customers and sell more belts.

Much of the focus of bogus devices was still on the bowels. "Dr. Young's Ideal Self-Retaining Rectal Dilators" were claimed to treat "dyspepsia, rheumatism, insomnia, asthma, disease caused by sluggish circulation, and malnutrition." Their use was claimed to be wonderful for women during pregnancy and menstruation. For men, they were particularly recommended for "prostate troubles." These types of devices were later coupled with electricity to make heated rectal probes that warmed the prostate internally.

Another scientific discovery that was ripe for medical fraud was invisible radiation. Scientists considered radium to have incredible amounts of energy locked up in its chemical atoms, so an illogical jump in reasoning by the medical quacks was that this energy could be transferred to humans by ingesting radium ore or radium water. After the discovery of radiation, radioactive material soon found its way into patent medicines, and a craze developed for drinking radium water.

Radium water, like electric treatments, was felt to carry energy into the core of the body. Machines containing radium were sold to home users who wanted to irradiate their tap water to make a home cure. Typical recommendations were to drink five or six glasses of radium water a day for sixty to ninety days in order to get the full benefit of the energy and eliminate disease.

Again, much of the focus was on the bowels. A typical consumer testimonial came from J.D. Bright of Silver City,

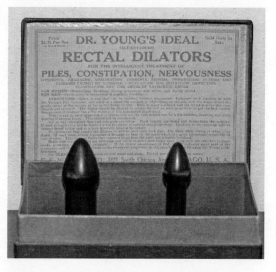

Many odd medical devices appeared during the golden age of patent medicines, including these devices that claimed to cure (among other diseases) asthma, malnutrition, and skin problems (author's collection).

New Mexico, who complained, "My stomach and bowels seemed deranged and I was constipated, had no appetite and felt bad all the time." After drinking radium water he delightedly said, "I have improved from the first day that I began drinking the water and gained six pounds in weight. Appetite is fine and constipation is cured. My digestion is now perfect and I am sleeping sound."[14] Old-timer Franklin Ford complained of rheumatism and feeling bad, but after drinking the same radium water he claimed he could jump up and pop his heels together.

Radioactive ore was added to other "health" products. In Grant County, New Mexico, Ra-Tor Mining and Manufacturing Company sold salves, toothpaste, and beauty products that were loaded with radium. As the dangers of radioactive material were realized, these products eventually left the market or were banned from medicines and personal products.

One of the odder cures that was heavily promoted was a craze for blue glass. When doctors claimed that wearing blue-tinted eyeglasses would cure every ailment, people started wearing tinted glasses, and even replaced the windows in their houses with blue glass. Hotels replaced their clear plate-glass windows with blue glass, and streetcars in the big cities installed blue glass in their horse-drawn cars. Like other fads, this one also faded away.[15]

CHAPTER ELEVEN

Dental and Eye Care

Dentistry

Estimates place the number of dentists in the entire United States in 1830 at about 300. By 1860 this number had grown to about 5,500 dentists. Almost all of these, however, were located on the East Coast. Dentists weren't common in small towns, particularly in the West, because more lucrative practices could be established in the bigger cities and in the East. With the lack of dentists in frontier towns, doctors were often also called upon to practice dentistry.

Dentistry was a relative late-comer among the healing arts. In 1881 there were only fifteen dental schools in the United States. With such a dearth of dental schools, dentists, like doctors, learned their profession by apprenticeship. The American Society of Dental Surgeons was established in 1840. By 1884 there were 103 dental societies around the country.

Dental hygiene on the early frontier was either poor or non-existent, and preventative measures, such as brushing and cleaning, were rarely practiced. Chewing wood charcoal once or twice a week was recommended for purifying bad breath and at the same time preserving teeth from decay. Some contemporary ideas about dental hygiene were peculiar, to say the least. For example, there was the belief that rinsing the mouth with one's own urine would eliminate bad breath and preserve the teeth. Bad dental hygiene allowed various infections to invade the gums and mouth. Blood poisoning occurring in the mouth was known as "black tongue."

Typically, little attention was given to the teeth until something went wrong with one of them. The outcome was usually that the offending tooth had to be pulled as a result of tooth decay. Due to a lack of medical knowledge and understanding of disease processes, rheumatism, stomach ailments, and fevers were sometimes "cured" by extracting decayed teeth.

A crude type of toothpaste made from soap was available by the late 1850s, but it was seldom used. As a result, most people had no teeth left by the time they reached the age of fifty. The absence of the four front incisors was a cause for rejection from the army. Before metallic cartridges were developed, soldiers tore open the tops of paper cartridges with their teeth. Missing front teeth meant that they could not accomplish this task. The lack of these four front teeth was abbreviated on military physical examination records as "4F," a designation that eventually became the category of exemption from military service for any physical disability.

Dentistry in the Old West was primitive, and the limited dental care that was available consisted primarily of tooth extraction. The cost was twenty-five to fifty cents per tooth. The alternatives for a man with a toothache were to do nothing and put up with the toothache, or to go to the dentist and have the tooth pulled out. Neither approach was appealing. If an extraction was performed poorly, the patient might be left with lacerated gums, a splintered jawbone, and more pain than he had previously.

If a dentist was available, tooth extraction was often performed in the patient's home. The absence of a dentist might make for an even more primitive cure. A man named Gus Grames, who lived in the mountains of Col-

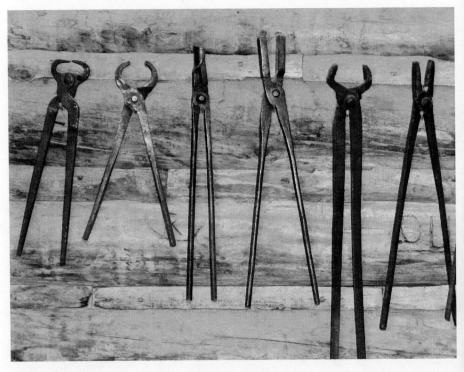

If no dentist was available, a blacksmith could use tools like these to pull an aching tooth (author's collection).

orado, suffered from a sudden toothache. His jaw swelled up, and by evening he was in severe pain. His partner had no surgical instruments, so he tried to pull out the offending tooth with an old pair of hand-operated bullet molds. The jaws of the mold kept slipping off the tooth, so finally, not knowing what else to do, his partner knocked out the tooth with a spike and a hammer.

If a person was in agony from an aching tooth, and no other option was available, in desperation he might go to the local blacksmith, who had pliers and pincers that could be used to perform an extraction.

If a tooth was not too far gone with decay and could still be saved, dentists drilled out the cavity and inserted a filling made from gold foil, held in place by a creosote material. If a cowboy did not want a filling material as expensive as gold, tin foil could be substituted. An amalgam of silver, tin, and mercury was also used for fillings. A tooth that was merely broken might have the rough edges removed with a metal file or even a piece of sandpaper.

A small town in the middle of nowhere, or a remote mining camp, often did not have a regular dentist, but might be visited occasionally by a traveling dentist who journeyed around a regular circuit of small towns and outlying areas. These itinerant dentists set up a temporary office in a local hotel or in the back of a saloon and extracted teeth that had gone bad since their last visit.

Typical of early dentists in the Mountain West was W.H. Folsom, who opened an office in Durango, Colorado, in 1881 in the First National Bank Building. Even though the town had grown to 3,000 inhabitants since its founding in 1880, Folsom was the first dentist to move there. He treated his patients in a kitchen chair that had a home-made headrest. The entire contraption was mounted on a packing crate so that it was high enough for him to work conveniently. He also rode on horseback to the town of Silverton, fifty miles to the north through the mountains, to treat the men from the neighboring mines.

Dentist Henry Rose arrived in the mining town of Leadville in the summer of 1878 but was not able to find an office for the first three months he was there. So he treated his patients in a folding chair on the sidewalk at the corner of Chestnut Street and Harrison Avenue. The miners worked during the day, so his business hours were from six o'clock in the evening to ten o'clock. He used a kerosene lamp to provide enough light to see to work. Whiskey served double duty for sterilization and as an anesthetic.

The first woman to be licensed as a dentist in the Old West was Nellie Pooler Chapman, who qualified in 1879. She and her husband, also a dentist, practiced in Nevada City, California. Her husband, Allen, was so confident of her capabilities that he spent much of his time working their mining claim in Virginia City, Nevada, while she attended to the patients in California.

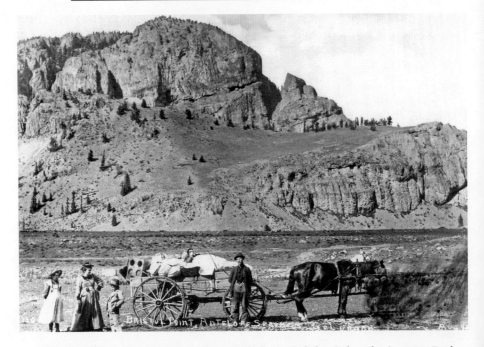

Dr. Howell D. Newton moved from Indiana to Salida, Colorado, in 1892. Each spring he loaded a secondhand barber's chair and his dental tools into a wagon, and went through the San Luis Valley to the San Juan Mountains, serving as an itinerant dentist. He worked his way back to Salida in the fall. Here he is seen with his wife and children at Bristol Point, Antelope Park, on August 15, 1895 (Special Collections, Tutt Library, Colorado College, Colorado Springs).

Even though soldiers at frontier posts during the Indian Wars had some of the best surgeons and medical care in the West at the time, they did not have dentists or routine dental care. The Military Dental Corps was not formed until 1901. As with other tooth sufferers on the frontier, treatment of tooth problems for soldiers was generally limited to the post surgeon pulling a decayed tooth when it caused enough pain. Military surgeons were not trained as dentists, so their limited attempts at treatment might leave a patient with a bad tooth in worse condition than he had been before.

Cowboys and miners viewed visits to the dentist with mixed emotions. Prospective patients knew that pain was usually involved in a dental visit, so they often delayed treatment, thinking to avoid it. By the time that increasing tooth pain made a visit unavoidable, it was usually too late. Because of the delayed treatment, the tooth decay continued, the pain became worse, and the tooth had to be pulled.

Cowboys, miners, and soldiers who hated the thought of the upcoming pain of having a tooth pulled often used an impending visit to the dentist as an excuse to drink large amounts of whiskey. They drank before the extraction to dull the inevitable pain, and afterwards to dull the residual ache from the visit.

Part of the problem of dentistry on the frontier was that the patient couldn't always tell which specific tooth was causing the pain. Because practitioners had to rely on the patient to tell them which tooth was causing problems, it was not unusual for the dentist to pull the wrong one. A dentist had to be a fast talker to explain this error. One apocryphal story concerns the time when notorious gunman Clay Allison went to a dentist in Cheyenne, Wyoming, in 1886 to have a tooth pulled. Supposedly, the dentist started working on the wrong tooth. The furious Allison went to another dentist to have the damage repaired, then in retaliation he went back and pulled out one of the first dentist's teeth. He started similar work on another tooth when the dentist's cries attracted a crowd and Allison was stopped.

Arguably the most famous dentist in the Old West was the tubercular Doc Holliday. He practiced dentistry briefly in Dallas and then Dodge City, but preferred gambling and showed up in almost every gambling town in the West. As his disease progressed, he often drank a quart of whiskey a day to dull the pain. Though he gained a reputation as a gunman, he probably did not kill as many men as he is credited for.

Dental Instruments

The basic dental implement was a good pair of plier-like forceps with which to yank out aching teeth. Another important instrument was the toothkey, a T-shaped device that hooked around a tooth and was then pushed upwards to extract the entire tooth. At least that was the theory. The result of this violent maneuver was that often a rotten tooth broke off at the gum line, and the remaining pieces had to be gouged out of the socket with a dental elevator, a device that looked like a small chisel. The use of a toothkey also sometimes broke the patient's jaw, which left him or her in more pain than before.

Various specialized designs of dental instruments included forceps intended for extracting specific teeth. Other specialized forceps,

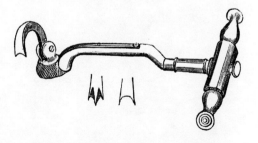

The dental implement that probably received the most use was the toothkey. The dentist hooked the curved end (at left) around the bad tooth and then pulled on the wooden handle on the right. Hopefully the tooth came out in its entirety with the first tug, but sometime it didn't (National Library of Medicine).

with curved gripping surfaces, were used for extracting fragments of teeth left by the tooth key, and for stumps of teeth that had rotted beyond the ability of simple removal. Scaling instruments for removing a build-up of tartar and other debris were available.

Dental instruments were treated with as much care as other contemporary surgical instruments and might be piled in a heap by the dental chair

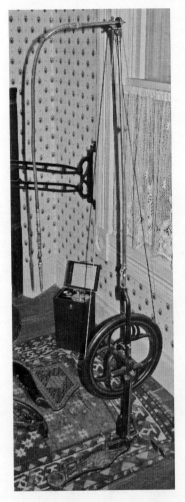

without being washed or sterilized between patients. The first dental tools were made with wooden handles— simply because handles on all sorts of tools had traditionally been made from wood. When the practice of sterilization of dental instruments became commonplace, instrument manufacturers realized that wooden handles would not withstand the process, and dental tools were constructed completely from metal.

Early dental drills were hand tools that gouged out tooth decay more than drilled it out. The dental drill turned by a flexible cable was introduced by Charles Merry of St. Louis in 1858. This device was powered by the dentist's foot pumping up and down on a pedal that operated a pulley to drive a belt to turn the drill bit. The bit rotated relatively slowly, making progress of the drilling very tedious and transmitting low vibrations through the patient's jaw to the rest of his head, creating a dull, grinding sound. This was accompanied by the smell of burning tooth enamel due to heat created by the slow cutting action of the drill bit. The lack of local anesthetics to dull the nerve in the tooth being drilled made the whole procedure very painful.[1] Today's dental drills operate at high speed, cutting fast without the accompanying dull, throbbing vibrations in the skull.

Early dental drills were powered by the dentist pumping a foot treadle. These drills were slow in speed and painful for the patient (author's collection).

Dental Anesthesia

Dental patients did indeed have something to worry about when they went to visit the dentist. Before anesthetics were introduced, the dentist often physically held his patient down in the

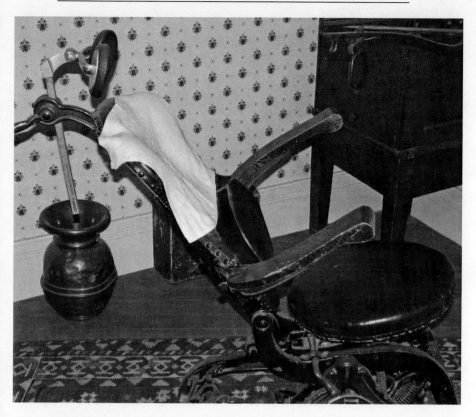

Frontier dentist's chairs were functionally not very different from those of today (author's collection).

chair with a knee on the chest while he yanked, pried, and twisted a bad tooth out of its socket as best he could. This was not always an easy task for a dentist to perform while his patient squirmed beneath him and groaned through a mouthful of instruments. The introduction of ether and nitrous oxide as anesthetics in dentistry in the early 1840s eliminated these crude procedures, making the process easier for both patient and dentist. One alternative, before gas anesthesia was developed, was to put opium or cocaine into the cavity of a decayed tooth in order to dull the nerve before extraction.

Several drugs could be applied to an aching tooth to temporarily dull the pain. One was cajuput oil, which was made from the leaves of the *melaleuca leucadendron* tree from Indonesia. A few drops, mixed with sugar, was also used to relieve spasms of the stomach and bowels. Ginger and mustard, made into poultices and applied to the cheek, were employed to relieve the pain of a toothache. What must have been the ultimate remedy for toothache was a mixture of sassafras oil, oil of cloves, summer-savory oil, and oil of cedar. The combination was applied to the tooth with a piece of lint. This must have been a powerful combination indeed, because all of these ingredients could be used separately to achieve the same purpose.

False Teeth

After decayed teeth were pulled out, replacement teeth were important, both for cosmetic reasons and to restore lost function. A set of false teeth in the Old West cost about eight dollars. Early tooth replacements were made from carved bone, ivory, or even natural animal or human teeth. Some early false teeth were made from hippopotamus or elephant tusks, which were a form of modified animal teeth.

For dentures to fit correctly, all of the old teeth had to be pulled, which was a horrible procedure to contemplate. Patients consumed copious amounts of whiskey, wine, or laudanum to dull the pain and the subsequent aching of the jaw, but it was still a very painful process.

Before proper techniques for installing dentures were developed, false teeth were glued to the remaining roots of the patient's own teeth. It later developed that this procedure was not particularly successful. The remaining root of the tooth continued to decay in the jaw, and the glue used to hold the false teeth in place discolored or turned black. With continued improvement of techniques, dentists learned how to extract the entire tooth in order to prevent further decay.

The development of the vulcanization of natural rubber by Charles Goodyear in 1839 led to the use of vulcanite (hard rubber) for dentures.[2] Dentists, noting the use of celluloid (a plastic based on cellulose nitrate) for billiard balls by J. Smith Hyatt in 1869, quickly adapted the same material for dentures.

The second half of the nineteenth century saw the development of improved false teeth that were made from porcelain, which was a mixture of the minerals feldspar, quartz, and clay. These ingredients were baked at high temperature to form a hard, impervious material that was ideal for dentures.

Eye Care

Not to slight the care of vision, which was very important, eye care in the Old West was limited due to the lack of techniques and instruments to safely operate on such a delicate organ. Specialists in the big cities could perform surgery to remove cataracts and carry out other procedures, but the frontier doctor had neither the training nor facilities to do the same.

Physicians did the best that they could with eyes that were injured through blunt trauma due to fights or industrial accidents. This often necessitated the careful removal of foreign objects that had been driven into the eyes. The removal of cinders from the eyes of railroad engineers and firemen was common. Some eye surgery was performed to remove other foreign objects that had become embedded in the eye; however, without the modern techniques of microsurgery, these efforts were limited. The instruments of the frontier doctor were limited mostly to various appliances to grasp the eyelid and retract it in order to extract foreign objects.

Patients frequently needed treatment for eyes that became inflamed or irritated by foreign objects, such as blown dirt in sandstorms, or for snow blindness. A common treatment was the use of boric acid-based eye drops to clear the irritation. Various other eyewashes, often compounded as home remedies, were also utilized. Most were reasonably conventional and benign, such as solutions derived from sassafras, blue violets, witch hazel, rosewater, ordinary tea, or a combination of hyssop leaves and

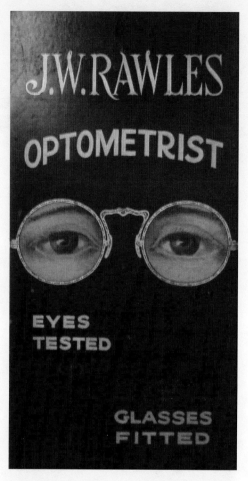

Elaborate sign for an optometrist who practiced in Pueblo, Colorado (author's collection).

St. John's wort leaves and flowers. An eyewash made from chamomile tea (from the aster family) was popular. A lead acetate solution (made from Goulard's powder) was also employed as an eyewash. One home remedy that was said to work quite well in an emergency was an eyewash made from gunpowder dissolved in water. Another folk remedy to soothe eye irritation was an extract of red willow bark in water, mixed with a little brandy. One of the more unusual treatments suggested for inflamed eyes was to split open a rotten apple and place the two halves over the eyelids to provide a cooling effect.

One interesting folk ointment that was good for sore eyes was the garden herb celandine mixed with butter and simmered for twelve hours, then

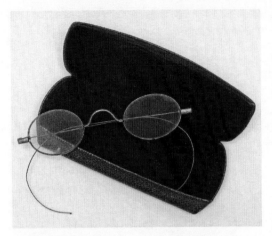

Though not as trendsetting as today's designs, the use of eyeglasses, such as these antique ones, for the correction of vision was the commonest type of eye treatment (author's collection).

applied as an ointment. In line with the practice of making the most economical use of folk remedies, this ointment was also recommended for hemorrhoids.

A significant advance in the examination of eyes occurred in 1851 when German physiologist (later to become a distinguished physicist) Hermann von Helmholtz developed the ophthalmoscope. His device allowed enough light to be projected into the eye for doctors to examine the blood vessels at the back of the eye for disease. Doctors had previously used a

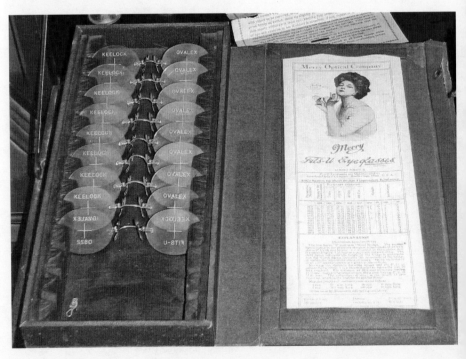

This set of eye lenses was used to determine the patient's prescription in the doctor's office (author's collection).

magnifying glass to look inside the eye but were not able to see much because of the inability to send in light and see inside at the same time. Von Helmholtz's new device allowed them to clearly examine the blood vessels on the retina.

A more advanced skill was optometry. Eyeglasses were available for refractive correction of far- and near-sightedness. Testing was limited to trying different lenses to see which one made the eyesight clearer.

CHAPTER TWELVE

American Indian Healing

The American Indian population of the Old West consisted of many different tribes scattered over different geographical and climatological areas, from the Canadian border to Mexico, and the Mississippi to the Pacific Coast. Many of the larger Indian tribes were concentrated over the Great Plains of the Midwest, the Rocky Mountains, and the deserts of the Southwest. Most of these tribes had different cultures, different ideas, and different languages. Such differences make it difficult to summarize the many approaches to natural healing that existed; thus, the following brief description will outline only the basics of Indian medicine.

Before the arrival of the white men — trappers, soldiers, miners, farmers, and other settlers — diseases were not typically rampant among Native American Indians, and they enjoyed relatively good health. The Indians generally led a relatively sanitary lifestyle in the outdoors. Most Indians bathed frequently and kept themselves clean, and were usually much cleaner than many of the white miners, cowboys, and prospectors. Their cooking and eating habits involved clean practices, and many of the gastrointestinal diseases suffered by the whites, such as cholera and typhoid, did not fester and spread among them. Nomadic tribes packed up periodically and moved to a new, clean camp, leaving behind them any accumulated trash and filth, and the areas used for individual toilet facilities.

A lifestyle of fresh air, fresh water, and clean food allowed the Indians to avoid many of the disease problems of the whites, who were often crowded together in close quarters in a city, town, or wagon train on the move westwards.

The main medical issue that the Indians had to face before the arrival of the whites was injury sustained during the hunt for food, or during raids or fights with neighboring tribes. Native American Indians had to contend with many of the same injuries as the white man. Broken bones, dislocated joints, sprained muscles, and wounds were the hazards of being a young Indian male. Other complaints were stomach upsets from a poor diet during the winter and improperly-cooked food. Snakebites, skin rashes, and upper respiratory complaints, such as winter colds and coughs, were common. Influenza, particularly devastating to the susceptible native population, did not arrive until the white man came to the West.

Older Indians on the Great Plains and in the Rocky Mountains commonly suffered from arthritic complaints due to sleeping on the ground and from the harsh winters that descended on them for much of the year. The Ute Indians of the central Colorado mountains, for example, bathed in the local natural hot springs around Manitou Springs, Glenwood Springs, and Chalk Creek, near Buena Vista, for relief from aching battle wounds and rheumatic complaints.

The Spiritual Perspective on Healing

The world of the American Indian was dominated by spirituality. The Indians of the Old West believed that everything in the world around them was filled with unseen mystical powers and spirits that affected and con-

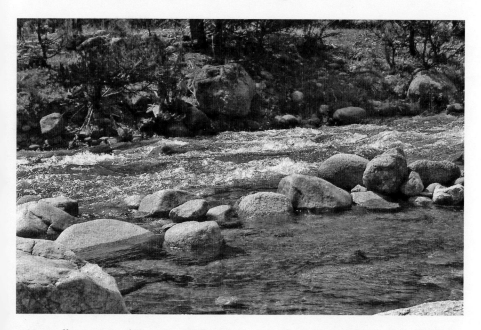

Naturally occurring hot springs and pools were used by American Indians to soothe away aches and pains, and as a treatment for battle wounds. This is Chalk Creek in central Colorado, where scalding hot underground springs mix with cool river water in creekside pools (foreground) to provide a comfortable temperature for bathing and soaking (author's collection).

trolled every aspect of their daily lives. These spirits were a part of each visible object and animal, and were often personified as the sun, earth, and moon. Other spirits controlled phenomena in the natural world around them, such as floods or eclipses.

The Indians believed that in order to survive, and for continued well-being and prosperity, they had to continually appease these unseen spirits through a series of rituals. Some were simple daily rituals. Others were manifested in complex dances and ceremonies. The spirits could either bring successes, such as protecting the tribe, or could plague the tribe with disaster, such as a scarcity of food or a poor hunting season. One way that diseases were contracted was thought to be through the neglect of these rituals. One belief, for example, was that severe arthritis was the result of not asking pardon of a deer for having to hunt and kill it for food and clothing materials.

Good health was part of this complex spiritual scheme. Virtually all the tribes believed that sickness and disease emerged in a person when the spirits were angry. As a result, one way to cure disease was to placate the offended spirits through spiritual rites. This was achieved through song, prayer, and ritualistic dances. The mediator between the sick person and the spirits was

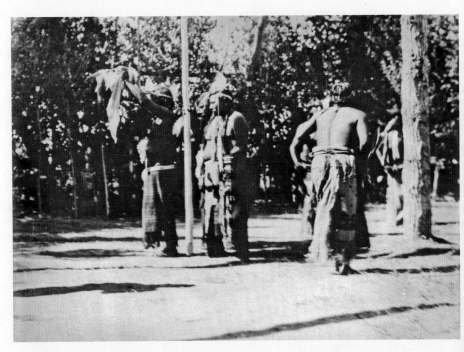

Sun Dance performed by an unidentified Plains Indian tribe in the late 1800s. These shamans are making "good medicine" (Denver Public Library Western History Collection, X-31946).

the medicine man, also known as a shaman. Medicine men were generally honored leaders among the tribe, often second only to the chief of the tribe, and were sought out for advice on many matters. Through religious dances, chants, and incantations the medicine man was able to intercede with the spirits on behalf of the ill individual. Herbal remedies were used to assist the healing process.

Another healing method employed by some of the Indians of the Southwest, such as the Navajo, was the curative value of sand paintings. These "paintings" started with a base layer of sand on the floor, then colored pigments derived from plant roots, charcoal, and pollens were trickled over the sand to form various designs as a type of dry painting. The paintings ranged in size from a foot to over twenty feet in diameter and contained symbolic representations of various religious features. After suitable incantations, the patient was placed in the middle of the painting, and further chants were performed to drive out of the patient's body the evil spirits causing the illness. After the ceremony, the design was erased and the sand brushed up in order to keep the specifics of the sacred paintings secret.

Though most medicine men were male, some tribes had female medicine "men." Among the Hupas, who lived in a remote area of northwest California, the healers were women. Women were also allowed to become medicine "men" among the Gros Ventre and the Crow tribes of Montana. In some cultures, women were not allowed to practice healing until after menopause because of the religious fear of menstruation.

As a rather drastic step among some Indian tribes, if the medicine man failed to save and cure his patient, the relatives of the deceased were allowed to kill the medicine man in retaliation.

The Medicine Man

Though medicine men existed in each Western tribe, their role and function was not always the same from tribe to tribe. Many of the shamans had diverse roles, such as performing rituals at major ceremonies, foretelling the future, attracting good weather, or bringing success for the hunt or a raid on a neighboring tribe. The shaman was primarily a ceremonial priest, but also served as the tribal healer to treat illness among the tribesmen. Some of these medicine men specialized in different areas of healing, such as treating battle wounds, setting broken bones, or curing diseases.

In the case of external disease or physical injury, the cause was generally obvious—as was the treatment, such as cleaning and binding an arrow wound in the flesh. Disease of an internal nature, such as smallpox or cholera, could not be seen, and the causes were attributed to the spirits invading the patient. While herbal medicines were used as part of the cure, more often the treatment was to try and drive out the offending spirit by rituals, charms, and incantations. The Cherokee, for example, recognized several dozen spirits that could cause diseases. It was the task of the medicine man to figure out which one was causing the problem and devise a "cure" for it. Among other cures to drive out spirits causing disease, the patient might be given foul-tasting medicine or an emetic to try and offend them and expel them. Purgative herbal medicines or enemas were also used to flush out these malignant spirits.

One belief that Indian medicine men held in common with white doctors of the mid-to-late nineteenth century was that much of sickness originated in the gastrointestinal tract. Therefore, similar to white doctors, one approach to healing was that "impurities" could be expelled from the upper gastrointestinal tract by emetics, or from the lower part of the system by purges or enemas. Following this, healing and soothing herbs were given as teas or similar medicines until the patient recovered. Because some gastric

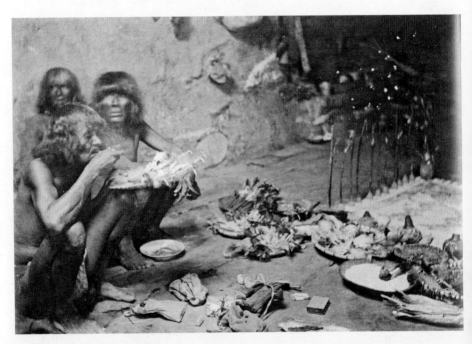

Hopi medicine men, surrounded by objects important to ritual ceremonies, inside a cave in Northern Arizona around 1899. A sand painting is on the floor next to them. Many of the Pueblo Indians had strong spiritual ties to caves, as they believed that the tribes emerged from below the surface of the earth in ancient times. Ceremonies performed in caves brought them closer to the supernatural spirits of the world below (Denver Public Library Western History Collection, X-30781).

illnesses and upsets arose from eating improperly cooked food and from parasites, this approach may have been effective for many stomach complaints.

The medicine man had several other means at his disposal. For the spiritual side of healing, a medicine pouch contained healing herbs and sacred talismans, amulets, and charms. For more practical cures, knives were used for primitive surgery or to lance boils and abscesses, and leather or wooden splints were utilized to bind up broken bones. Most medicine men had a mortar and pestle for crushing plant parts to make herbal medicines. A hollow tube, made from a bone and attached to a flexible animal bladder, was used as a primitive syringe for enemas or to administer medicines to irrigate wounds.[1] Similar bone tubes were used for sucking to relieve pus, remove excess blood, and to suck out the poison of snakebite or scorpion stings.

Among the medicine man's medical instruments might be a device for performing bleeding. Usually this was a crude knife made from obsidian or flint, though later replaced by iron or steel traded from the white man. It is uncertain whether the practice of bleeding was learned from the white man after his arrival in the West or whether it came up from the south, from other cultures such as Aztec medicine men, who bled their patients to relieve headaches, fever, and swelling.

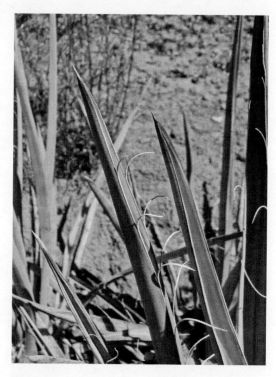

Wounds were sewn up with thread and a sharpened deer tendon. Thread was sometimes made from vegetable fiber, such as the long, spiny leaves of the yucca plant. The leaf fibers from the plantain were also employed for thread for sewing up wounds—the same thread used to make clothing or sew deer hide into moccasins. The yucca plant, however, wasn't always utilized for healing. The Navajo Indians mixed the juice squeezed from the leaves of the yucca

The sharp spine on the ends of the leaves of the yucca plant, which grew in many places in the West, was used as a needle, and the stringy fibers of the leaves were used as thread to sew up wounds. The root of the yucca was used to make soap (author's collection).

plant with rattlesnake blood to make a potent poison with which they coated their arrows for battle.

Some medicine men specialized in the treatment of arrow and bullet wounds, a skill that was important after fights between warring tribes and during the Indian Wars in the West of the second half of the nineteenth century. The technique was similar to that practiced by white doctors, though the tools were more primitive. Instead of a metal probe and surgical bullet forceps, the medicine man might use a split willow stick inserted into the wound. After locating the arrowhead or bullet, the two halves of the stick were squeezed together to hold the object while it was being withdrawn.

Sweatbaths in special lodges were used for ritual purification of illnesses. In a more practical sense, the heat generated in this process certainly had curative value for aches and pains. The commonest type of sweat lodge consisted of a circle of willow saplings bent over to the ground to form a framework, with a buffalo hide roof stretched over the top. Steam was generated by sprinkling water over rocks heated in a firepit in the middle of the lodge. Herbs were sometimes added to the water to make a medicated steam to increase the medicinal effect.

These sweat lodges were remarkably similar to the vapor baths employed by conventional medicine among the white settlers. This technique was used to provide heat to a patient in cases of rheumatism, fevers, and other treatments. The recommended procedure was to make a frame and cover it with canvas. The patient stood or sat in this enclosure while steam was introduced into it from a boiler on a nearby fireplace. This device and process allowed the patient to work up a good sweat.

Medicinal Herbs

The Indian medicine men were able to cope fairly well with minor illnesses. Over many generations they had developed a collection of medicines, based on plant life, that provided empirical cures. A comparison shows that many of the Indian cures were similar to the pioneers' folk medicine; indeed, many pioneer cures were derived from Indian medicines. Many of the same plants were also used for food, including the bitterroot, biscuitroot, camas, wild lily, cattail, and burrweed.

Roots, barks, and flowering plants were utilized to make medicines and teas that accompanied the spiritual part of the healing process. The leaves and twigs of the Oregon grape, for example, were used by the Navajo to treat rheumatism. The gray-blue berries of the Utah juniper were employed to treat urinary infections.

One general concept stated that curative medicines were similar to the disease being cured. This was called the "doctrine of signatures" and meant that plants used for treatment had the shape or color of the body part being treated. Red plants, for example, were used to treat blood disorders, and yellow plants were utilized to treat yellowing diseases, such as jaundice. Plants might also be used for medicines because they resembled the body part being treated. These principles were not always followed, though, as certain plants were known through long association to be effective in treating particular diseases.

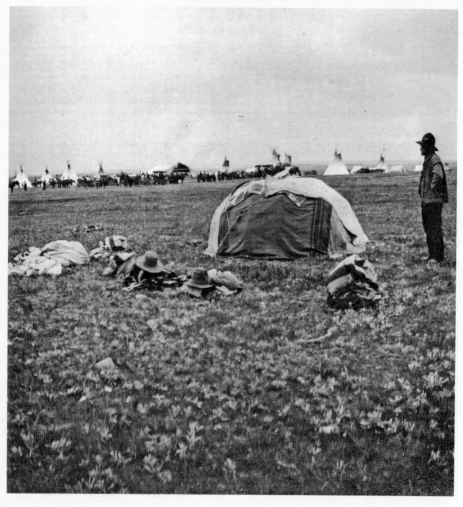

Native American (Blackfoot) sweat lodge on the open plains of Montana around 1900. The piles of clothing outside the structure indicate that it was in use (Denver Public Library Western History Collection, X-31131).

Some herbal concoctions had other uses. For example, some Indian tribes believed that death camas would keep away evil spirits if the plant was placed around their camps.

Many plant cures had legitimate medicinal properties. Willow bark and the bark of the aspen tree, for example, contained a substance similar to aspirin that was used to soothe minor aches and treat fever. Soothing teas were made from a variety of plants, including the long-plumed avens, chokecherry, spirea, gumweed, coneflower, and prince's pine. Tea made from the Oregon grape was employed to cleanse the blood and treat anemia. Tea made from the skunkbush was used to treat ulcers and cuts. A tea made from the stems of the plant was utilized to soothe coughs. Chewing gum was made from the dried juice of the hawkweed, false dandelion, and pussytoes.

Herbal medicines were applied in a number of ways. Plants, roots, flowers, seeds, and bark might be crushed and boiled to extract the medicinal element in liquid form. Another approach was to use these same ingredients to make a tea. The resulting medicine could be drunk, poured on a wound, or injected as an enema. Though the commonest route of administration was via the mouth, some herbal remedies could not be tolerated when taken orally, and were given via the rectum. One example was meadowsweet (from the rose family). It had properties similar to aspirin, but it was not edible, so it was administered as an enema. It relieved pain, inflammation, and stomach disorders. Blackfoot Indian women also used it as a douche to treat various forms of venereal disease. The Blackfeet used the pasqueflower (part of the buttercup family) to speed up childbirth, or in large doses to deliberately induce miscarriage.

When mixed with bear or buffalo fat, herbal ingredients could be applied as a salve or poultice. Some leaves and other plant parts were smoked like tobacco to apply the medicine, such as for treating asthma or other lung-related diseases.

The Comanche used deadly nightshade (black nightshade) as a cure for tuberculosis. They had to be careful of the dosage, however. All the parts of the nightshade plant contains the poison solanine, and eating unripe berries could result in paralysis or death. The Pawnee ground up Indian turnips to make a cure for headaches. The Ute made a salve for cuts and bruises from the yarrow plant.[2] A tonic made from the plant was also useful as a stimulant. The Cheyenne used wild mint boiled in water to settle the stomach.

A bitter tonic was made from the mountain gentian. A medicine made from the root of the curlydock was used as a laxative and a tonic. The leaves of the clematis were chewed as a treatment for colds and sore throats. The juice of the salsify was used for indigestion. Arnica was utilized both to raise the body temperature and as a salve to reduce infection in wounds. Peyote was employed by the Apache in southern Arizona in the form of a poultice for fractures and snakebite. Peyote contained mescaline, which made it useful as a painkiller.

The Dakotas used the powdered roots of skunkcabbage to relieve asthma.[3] The roots of the skunkcabbage were also boiled, dried, and ground up to make a type of flour. Caution had to be exercised when gathering skunkcabbage because the toxic false hellebore (American hellebore, or poke root) grew in the same places and looked like skunkcabbage in the early spring. One way to tell the difference was that skunkcabbage, when crushed, had a very disagreeable smell, somewhat like its namesake the skunk. False hellebore was used in moderate doses by Indians to slow the heartbeat and lower blood pressure, though it was fatal if taken in large doses.

Medicine men of different tribes employed different medicines for the same purpose. The Cheyenne drank a tea made from the leaves and stems of a type of bloodroot for cramping in the bowels. The Ute used the sand puff, and the Oglala Sioux used the leaves of *Parosela aurea* for the same cure.

One reason for utilizing different medicinal herbs to treat the same condition was that the medicine man typically used what was available locally. The Apache of southern Arizona, for example, made poultices from the tops of the greasewood (chaparral or creosote bush) for the treatment of rheumatism because the bush was common in the area. The Plains Indians used the dried flowers of the false lupine for treatment of the same condition.

Venereal diseases were often treated by herbal means. One of the traditional Indian herbal cures for syphilis was to use the Indian tobacco plant to induce vomiting. Like many other "cures" for syphilis, this one may have seemed effective if the disease subsequently advanced into the latent phase. The Navajo used the root of the Oregon grape to treat syphilis and dysentery. The Comanche treated gonorrhea with a drink made from boiled thistle roots. A less pleasant treatment by the Crow involved placing hot rocks under the patient's genitals while the local medicine man threw herbal medicine at him.

Herbal medicines were also employed as aphrodisiacs. The Ojibwa Indians used lousewort for this purpose. The medicine acted as a mild irritant of the urinary tract, similar to the effect of Spanish Fly among whites, and made the user feel a sensation of arousal.

Tobacco also featured in the Indian pharmacopeia. One use was to induce vomiting to "purify" the body. There were other, less-enticing, uses for tobacco. Among the Cheyenne, a man who wanted to rekindle his wife's love rubbed a mixture of saliva and tobacco over her body while she was asleep, chanting magical incantations at the same time. Presumably he would have to perform this ceremony fast, before she woke up. The Creek Indians treated patients with stomach cramps by having them drink a potion of tobacco and water. Smoking materials were also made from a mixture of the dried leaves of the ground-hugging kinnikinnick plant and the inner bark of the dogwood.

Medicinal herbs were also used by the shamans themselves as a part of religious rituals. During the second half of the nineteenth century, the Apache, Navajo, Comanche, Kiowa, Sioux, and other Plains Indians used peyote for rituals that involved singing, chanting, meditation, and prayer. Peyote, which was derived from sacred cactus and contained the hallucinogenic drug mescaline, produced brilliantly-colored visions, similar to the later use of LSD (lysergic acid diethylamide). The drug was typically concocted as a drink made from the leaves and roots of the cactus plant. Because this brew could cause nausea and stomach upsets when taken by mouth, it was sometimes administered as an enema as part of the religious ritual. Peyote was also used medicinally by the shamans to treat arthritis, tuberculosis, influenza, and gastric problems among tribal members.

One of the ironies of Native American Indian medicine was that it later gained an almost mystical reputation for healing when incorporated into the craze for patent medicines. Manufacturers and salesman — white men, of course — promoted many of the medicines as being original Indian secret cures entrusted to them by medicine men.

Herbal plants had other, more sinister, uses than medicine. The roots of the Rocky Mountain iris were mixed with animal bile in a container made from an animal bladder, and warmed for several days. Arrows were dipped in the resulting mixture and used in battle. Reputedly, opponents that were even only slightly wounded died within a few days.

One of the more curious Indian herbal treatments was the use of stinging nettles. Contact with the leaves of stinging nettles caused skin irritation, pain, and itching due to hair-like filaments on the underside of the leaves that injected formic acid (the substance found in ant bites) into the skin. Indians sometimes beat themselves with these leaves as a treatment to relieve the swelling and pain of arthritis. One would presume that this produced the substitution of one type of pain for another.

A final interesting use of plants involved the employment of sage (from the mint family) to hasten the weaning of a suckling infant when the mother felt that the time was right. The woman drank large amounts of tea made from the sage plant, which gave the milk an undesirable flavor.

The White Man's Legacy

Unfortunately, the arrival of fur trappers, and later white settlers, brought with them a series of severe European diseases, such as smallpox, malaria, influenza, syphilis, and cholera, that spread rapidly among the Indians. These diseases were common among the whites, and probably of long standing due to the crowded conditions of European cities and the big cities of the East.[4] Not having been exposed to many of the common European diseases, the native Indian population had not developed any immunity and were highly susceptible to them. The effect of many of the relatively harmless childhood diseases on adults was often deadly.

The transmission of disease could be deadly in more ways than one. Marcus Whitman was a medical doctor and Presbyterian missionary who journeyed to the Pacific Northwest to establish a mission in the Walla Walla Valley to convert the Nez Perce and Cayuse tribes to Christianity. In his medical capacity, he treated members of the local tribes who became ill.

The Indians were not particularly receptive to his preaching and grew increasingly resentful of the horde of white settlers pouring into their territory. The final straw for the Indians was when a passing wagon train brought an epidemic of measles with it. Whitman tried to use his medical skills to cure the children of both the wagon train and the local Indians. The white children, many of whom had been previously exposed to the disease, mostly recovered. The Indian children, who had never been exposed and thus had no immunity, were decimated. The Cayuse believed that Whitman and his wife, Narcissa, were secretly poisoning the children with their medicines so that the white men could steal their land. Believing that the whites were responsible for the deaths of their children, several of the Cayuse, led by Chief Tiloukaikt, entered the mission and killed Whitman and his wife on November 29, 1847. Before the massacre was over, eleven others working at the mission had been slaughtered alongside them.

Afterword

Looking back at the state of medicine in the Old West from today's perspective, it is hard to imagine a time when diseases like smallpox and diphtheria could decimate a town, and one woman in ten who gave birth did not survive the experience. The end of the nineteenth century marked the beginning of discoveries and changes that resulted in major medical innovations to cure diseases and treat conditions that were deadly to pioneers in the Old West. Work that led to the discovery of insulin to control diabetes, which was then a fatal disease, took place in the early 1920s. The first sulfa drug (sulfanilimide) to combat previously deadly *Streptococcus* infections was developed in 1935. Sulfa drugs, which could heal many bacterial diseases, saved millions of lives and were the primary treatment for infectious diseases until the widespread use of penicillin in the late 1940s.

A true wonder drug, the penicillin mold (*Penicillium notatum*) was first discovered by accident in 1929 by Alexander Fleming. Fleming made a cursory investigation of the properties of the new substance but did not pursue its possible uses and turned to other interests. It was not until the late 1930s and early 1940s that other investigators realized the drug's potential for killing bacteria. Only during the last few years of World War II could enough penicillin be produced to treat servicemen wounded in battle. It was 1946 before penicillin became generally available to cure those afflicted with gonorrhea.

Tuberculosis was a major disease and killer in the Old West until the tuberculin test, a skin test to detect the infection, was developed. A combination of an improved standard of living, the use of x-rays for general screening of the population, and the development of the antibiotic streptomycin significantly lowered death rates from TB. Tuberculin testing of cattle and pasteurization of milk largely eliminated dairy products as a source of the disease. Ordinances against spitting in public helped curb its spread.

Wilhelm Konrad Roentgen discovered x-rays in 1895, at the very end of the nineteenth century. The use of these invisible rays allowed physicians to see inside the body to detect foreign objects and damaged organs, to look at broken bones, and to visualize the workings of the gastrointestinal tract. X-rays have proven to be invaluable to modern surgeons and are important in the treatment of cancer with radiation.

Even though the first half of the twentieth century was a time of rapid development of modern medicine and surgery, about 90 percent of the modern medical miracles that we take for granted today date from the end of World War II in 1945. The list of medical achievements is impressive. Heart, liver, and lung transplants are possible. Powerful new drugs combat cancer and AIDS. The human genome project has opened the way for advanced diagnosis and treatments. The development of machines for kidney dialysis has extended the life of people with failing kidneys until a transplant can be arranged. Oral contraceptives, first perfected in the 1950s, offer women precise control of family planning. By 1950, the average life expectancy for a man had risen to sixty-six years of age; for a woman, it had risen to seventy-three years.

Beyond the use of x-rays, several other radical new methods have been developed for imaging the inside of the human body. Ultrasonic imaging, which uses high frequency sound waves to see internal organs, is particularly useful for pregnant women when x-rays would harm the fetus. Thermography detects and analyzes minute temperature differences in tissue to detect cancer tumors and arthritic joints. Computer axial tomography (CAT) scanning combines x-rays with computer analysis to create a three-dimensional view of sections of the internal organs. Magnetic resonance imagining (MRI) uses a powerful magnetic field to excite hydrogen atoms in the body to create a three-dimensional image of soft tissues. Fiber optic endoscopes inserted into body openings allow a direct view of the inside of the gastrointestinal tract.

As we continue into the twenty-first century, medical developments that have not yet been thought of will continue to improve longevity and produce cures for diseases, such as cancer and AIDS, and age-related bodily degeneration, in ways that do not even seem possible today.

Glossary

There is a fine distinction between some closely-related medical terms. For example, there is a subtle difference between vaccination and inoculation. This glossary defines and explains some of these terms, with cross-references to similar, but different, terms. The following are not all-encompassing definitions, but are intended as explanations of some of the specialized medical terms that appear in the text. Some of the definitions are used in the context of nineteenth century medicine and may have slightly different meanings today.

Addiction: Domination by a drug habit.

Anesthetic: A local anesthetic (such as cocaine) blocks pain from a small area of the body while the patient is awake; a general anesthetic (such as ether) puts the patient to sleep.

Aperient: A very mild laxative. Derived from a Latin word meaning to "open" the bowels (see also *laxative*).

Arthritis: Inflammation of a joint due to various conditions; usually accompanied by pain in the joint.

Bacillus: A specific family of rod-shaped, disease-causing bacteria (see also *bacteria*, *rickettsia*, and *virus*).

Bacteria: One-celled living microorganisms that can produce disease in their host; bacteria can typically be killed in humans by antibiotics, or on surfaces by chemicals (disinfection) or the application of heat (see also *rickettsia* and *virus*).

Bilious: A symptom of a disordered liver, causing constipation, headache, and loss of appetite. The term was used as a catch-all name for any malaise by manufacturers of patent medicines.

Catarrh: An older generic medical term used to describe any inflammation of the mucus membranes of the breathing organs, such as in the throat and lungs.

Cathartic: A medicine that produces a series of violent bowel evacuations, often accompanied by pain and cramping (see also *laxative* and *purgative*).

Chlorosis: This nineteenth century term was often used interchangeably with "hysteria," a psychosomatic disease of women. The more modern meaning refers to a form of iron-deficiency anemia, particularly in young women. It was also called "green sickness" because the skin took on a greenish pallor. This form of chlorosis is not seen now because of modern nutrition (see also *hysteria*).

Clyster: An older medical term that generally referred to an enema, but the term clyster also included injections of healing substances into the ear, nose, bladder, and uterus. Older texts sometimes spell this as "glyster" (see also *enema* and *injection*).

Costiveness: An old fashioned term for constipation.

Diaphoretic: A medicine intended to promote sweating (see also *sudorific*).

Diarrhea: Abnormally frequent, uncontrolled evacuations of the bowel that are symptomatic of an intestinal disorder or infectious fever (see also *dysentery*).

Diuretic: A drug used to increase the excretion of urine.

Dropsy: An older term for the accumulation of fluid in the body due to congestive heart failure.

Dysentery: A name applied to a collection of intestinal diseases and disorders that cause diarrhea and are characterized by inflammation of the bowel wall (see also *diarrhea*).

Dyspepsia: Indigestion arising from various causes, such as disease, excessive use of alcohol, or dietary problems.

Emetic: A substance that produces vomiting.

Emmenagogue: An agent that stimulates menstrual flow.

Enema: An instrument or procedure for cleansing the colon or injecting medication into the bowels (see also *clyster* and *injection*).

Erisipelas: *Streptococcus* infection that causes fever and swelling of tissue under the skin. Also known as St. Anthony's Fire.

Felon: Inflammation at the end of a finger or toe. Also called a whitlow.

Fracture: A simple (closed) fracture is a broken bone covered by intact skin; a compound (open) fracture is a broken bone with a jagged end protruding through the skin; a comminuted or greenstick fracture is a splintered or crushed break in a bone that is covered by intact skin.

Greensickness: See *chlorosis*.

Grip or **grippe:** An older name for influenza.

Heroic Medicine: Medical treatments based on ancient humoral theory and consisting primarily of bleeding, purging, blistering, vomiting, and sweating to rebalance the humors.

Humoral Theory: Ancient Greek theory that there were four fluids, called humors, from which the body was thought to be composed: blood (sanguis), phlegm (pituita), yellow bile (chole), and black bile (melanchole). These corresponded to the four material elements of air, water, fire, and earth; and four conditions of hot, wet, cold, and dry. Good health depended on the balance of the four humors, and sickness meant that they were out of balance.

Hysteria: An imprecise diagnosis, derived from the Greek name for the womb, used to describe a series of nebulous symptoms in women that could be related to almost every type of physical disease. The condition was accompanied by various nervous and mental symptoms, such as laughing and crying for no reason, amnesia, tremors, vomiting, sleep-walking, limb paralysis, and psychotic episodes. Exhibition of these symptoms is now termed "hysterical neurosis" by psychotherapists (see also *neurasthenia, vapors,* and *chlorosis*).

Inoculation: Deliberate injection of a virus into an individual's body to prevent the acquisition of a specific disease, such as rabies or typhoid (see also *vaccination*).

Injection: Before the introduction of hypodermic injections under the skin, the term "injection" was used to describe an enema. "Throwing up an injection" was antique terminology for administering an enema.

Laceration: A cut or irregular tearing of the flesh.

Lancet: A sharp knife used for bleeding a patient. The leading British medical journal *The Lancet* is named after this instrument.

Laxative: A medicine that produces a mild bowel movement (see also *aperient, cathartic* and *purgative*).

Miasma: A foul and unpleasant exhalation or odor, typically from swampy areas, that was thought to be the cause of many diseases.

Neuralgia: Severe pain associated with a nerve.

Neurasthenia: A nebulous mental "disease" of men, with symptoms similar to hysteria in women, that showed symptoms of various diseases without any organic cause. It was accompanied by fatigue, weakness, irritability, an inability to concentrate, and various aches and pains (see also *hysteria, vapors,* and *chlorosis*).

Peritonitis: Inflammation of the peritoneum, which is the lining of the abdomen.

Phthisis: A wasting disease caused by lung problems. Miner's phthisis, for example, was a lung disease caused by inhaling rock dust in the mines. The term was commonly linked with various forms of tuberculosis.

Poultice: A hot, moist paste applied to the skin, then covered with a linen cloth or towel; used to relieve congestion or pain.

Pulmonary: Associated with the lungs.

Purgative: A medicine that causes violent action of the bowels to produce complete evacuation of the contents, usually accompanied by pain and severe cramping (see also *cathartic* and *laxative*).

Pus: Thick yellowish-green liquid that exudes from a wound, consisting of dead cells, decomposed tissue, bacteria, and liquid caused by inflammation.

Rheumatism: A general term applied to a series of acute and chronic complaints characterized by stiffness and soreness in the muscles and pain in the joints. This includes arthritis. See also *arthritis.*

Rickettsia: A group of organisms that are intermediate in size and complexity between a virus and a bacteria; the causative agent of many diseases, they are usually transmitted by vectors such as lice and fleas.

Septicemia: Blood poisoning.

Shock: Collapse due to circulatory failure, often due to a massive loss of blood from a wound.

Sterilization: The process of making surgical instruments or materials, such as hospital walls, free from living microorganisms that can cause disease.

Stomachic: Strengthening to the stomach, a medicine, like wine, that excited the action of the stomach.

Sudorific: A medicine intended to promote sweating; specifically an agent that causes drops of perspiration to appear on the skin (see also *diaphoretic*).

Tincture: A drug in a solution of 10 percent to 20 percent alcohol.

Tourniquet: A strap or other constricting device that is placed around an arm or leg to compress an artery or large vein to control bleeding, such as during an amputation procedure or after a major wound to an extremity.

Vaccination: Inoculation with a vaccine made from killed or weakened viruses and bacteria as a preventative measure against a specific disease (see also *inoculation*).

Vapors: An obsolete, vague term that applied to hysterical symptoms in women. It is now called hypochondriasis, and is applied to a situation where misinterpretation of physical symptoms by the patient leads to the belief that serious disease is present, even though medical evaluation can prove no physical basis (see also *hysteria*).

Vector: A carrier, often an insect such as a mosquito or flea, that transmits a disease from an infected individual to an uninfected one.

Virus: Minute infectious agent that reproduces within a host cell to cause disease, but is not killed by an antibiotic (see *bacteria* and *rickettsia*).

Whitlow: See *felon*.

Appendix A: Common Drugs, 1850–1900

Antimony: A poisonous heavy metal; used to produce purging and vomiting.

Arsenic: A highly poisonous metallic element in weed killers, insecticides, and rat poison; used as a treatment for syphilis. In small doses, arsenic was thought to strengthen the lungs and improve a woman's complexion.

Asafetida: A gum resin substance obtained from various perennial herbs; used as a medicine to relieve spasms.

Belladonna: Extracted from the leaves of the deadly nightshade plant (*Atropa belladonna*), the active ingredient is atropine; used to relieve pain, as a sedative for the stomach and bowels, to check perspiration, and to stimulate breathing.

Calomel: Mercurous chloride (chloride of mercury, also called horn mercury or sweet mercury); used for purging the bowels and treating syphilis.

Cantharides: A powder made from the dried and crushed body of the Spanish Fly, a large green beetle (*Cantharis vesicatoria*) that contained a substance that was highly irritating to the skin; used as a blistering agent.

Carbolic acid: Also known as phenol, a substance derived from the distillation of coal tar; used as a general disinfectant and as a douche by women to prevent venereal disease.

Castor oil: An unpleasant-tasting oil made from the beans of the castor plant (*Ricinus communis*); used as a laxative.

Chloroform: A liquid (methylene trichloride); used as a general anesthetic during surgery.

Cocaine: A drug obtained from the coca plant (*Erythroxylon coca*) that grew in Peru; used as a local anesthetic to dull pain in the skin.

Colocynth: The pulp of the fruit from the decorative plant *Citrullos colocynthis*; used as a drastic purgative.

Croton oil: An oil made from the ripe seeds of the croton plant (*Croton tiglium*) grown in Ceylon (now Sri Lanka) and China; used as a dramatic purgative.

Digitalis: An extract of the dried leaves of the foxglove plant (*Digitalis purpurae*); used as a heart stimulant. It also worked as a diuretic because it improved heart action and circulation.

Dover's powder: A mixture of opium, ipecac, and sugar of milk (lactose); used as a sedative or to produce sweating.

Epsom salts: Magnesium sulfate, named after the famous Epsom Spa in Surrey, England, whose water contained the salts; used as a laxative.

Ergot: Derived from a fungus (*Claviceps purpurea*) that grows on rye and some grasses; used to stimulate uterine contractions or to stop excessive bleeding after childbirth.

Ether: A gas (diethyl ether); used to produce anesthesia during surgery.

Fowler's solution: Named after Thomas Fowler, an English physician, this solution contained 1 percent arsenic trioxide (white arsenic), also known as potassium arsenite; used to treat nerve pain and muscular twitching.

Gamboge: gum resin of the *Garcinia norella* tree from India; used as a cathartic.

Glauber's salts: Sodium sulfate, named after German physician Johann Glauber, who first extracted the chemical from Hungarian spring water; used as a laxative.

Goulard's powder: Lead acetate (sugar of lead), named after Thomas Goulard, a French physician; used in solution externally for inflammatory conditions, such as sprains or bruises. Also used internally.

Heroin: Diacetyl morphine, a highly addictive narcotic derived from morphine; used for the treatment of asthma or a cough. The Narcotics Control Act of 1956 made the acquisition, possession, or transportation of heroin illegal.

Ipecac: Medicine derived from the dried roots of a South American creeping plant, *Cephaelis ipecacuanha*; used as an emetic, diaphoretic, and to treat amebic dysentery.

Jalap: Derived from the tuberous root of the Mexican plant *Convolvulus jalapa*; used as a strong purgative, with dramatic and explosive effects. Sometimes made more palatable by adding the required dosage to a cup of tea.

Laudanum: An alcohol solution of opium (tincture of opium); used as a sedative, a painkiller, and to check diarrhea.

Mercury: A heavy, poisonous metallic element that is liquid at room temperature; used medicinally primarily as calomel (mercurous chloride) as a purgative, but sometimes injected as a bead of liquid metal into the urethra to "cure" syphilis.

Morphine: One of the most important alkaloids derived from opium; used as a narcotic and to control severe pain.

Nitrous oxide: A gas that produces short periods of anesthesia; used for minor surgical procedures, such as extracting a tooth.

Opium: Made from the dried juice of the poppy plant *Papaver somniferum*, cultivated in the Far East, opium contains over twenty-five alkaloids that are used in medicine; opium and its medicinally important derivatives, laudanum and morphine, were prescribed for pain control and for ailments such as consumption, rheumatism, insomnia, and stomach disorders.

Paragoric: Tincture of opium with camphor; used to soothe teething babies and to check diarrhea.

Phenol: See *carbolic acid.*

Plummer's pills: A pill composed of antimony, jalap and calomel; used as a powerful purgative.

Quinine: Also known as Peruvian Bark or Jesuit Bark, quinine is a bitter substance derived from the bark of the *cinchona* family of trees that grow in South America; used primarily as a preventative for malaria, it was also employed to reduce fevers and relieve pain.

Rochelle salts: A combination of sodium tartarate and potassium tartarate; used as a laxative.

Spanish Fly: See *cantharides.*

Strychnine: A poisonous material derived from the seeds of the *Nux vomica* plant; used in small doses to stimulate the heart and breathing; also used as a tonic in debilitating diseases and to stimulate natural bowel function.

Tartar emetic: White, poisonous, metallic-tasting crystals of antimony and potassium tartarate; used as an emetic, sedative, counter-irritant, and sweating agent, especially for croup, colds, and fever. Other uses for women included treatment for difficult labor and painful breasts.

Whiskey: Ethyl alcohol (ethanol) with various colorings and flavorings; a beverage considered to be a universal cure for many ailments on the frontier, as well as an antiseptic and, in large enough quantities, an anesthetic. Whiskey was sometimes combined with quinine for the treatment or prevention of malaria.

Appendix B: Typical Surgical Instrument Kit

In 1850, the office of the surgeon-general of the Army provided an inventory of standard medical instruments for field use to military surgeons in the West. The following similar list is typical of instruments carried and used by physicians in the Old West.

Instrument	Use
Amputating instruments (various knives and saws)	Amputating limbs and extremities
Bougies (rubber and metal)	Slender metal or rubber tubular instruments for exploring and dilating body canals, such as the male urethra, the esophagus, the uterus, or the rectum
Catheters (rubber and metal)	Thin rubber or silver tubes typically used for draining the bladder or injecting medicine
Cupping glasses	Small glass cups placed over cuts to promote the flow of blood during bleeding procedures
Dental instruments	Pliers and tooth-keys for extracting teeth
Forceps, various types	Clamping bleeding veins and arteries; extracting bullets and arrow heads
Lancets (also known as fleams)	Bleeding
Obstetrical instruments	Childbirth
Probes	Slender metal rods for finding bullets or arrowheads embedded in flesh
Scarificator	Special knives with four to sixteen blades for bleeding procedures
Splints, assorted	To immobilize broken legs and arms

Stethoscope	For listening to the heart, lungs, and bowel sounds
Surgeon's needle and thread	Sewing up wounds
Syringe, enema	To cleanse the bowels or inject medicine
Syringe, penis	Injecting medicine into the urethra for treating venereal disease
Tourniquets	To stop blood flow during amputation or in case of severe bleeding in legs and arms
Trepanning instruments	Operating on skull fractures
Trusses	Supporting hernias

Emetics included in the physician's black bag typically included alum, ipecac, mustard, tartar emetic, and zinc sulfate. Purgatives included aloes, calomel, castor oil, Epsom salt, jalap, rhubarb, and senna. A small amount of quinine was included for treating malaria.

List adapted from Hall, *Medicine on the Santa Fe Trail*, 75.

Notes

Chapter One

1. Hertzler, *The Horse and Buggy Doctor*, 34.

2. These techniques were of long-standing use in Europe. In the Middle Ages, bleeding, the use of clysters (enemas), and blistering were common medical practices. These treatments were usually administered by barber-surgeons because European physicians of the time thought that performing such duties was beneath their dignity. In the seventeenth century in France, King Louis XIII is estimated to have undergone 47 bleedings, 215 purges, and 212 enema treatments in a single year.

3. During his final illness, President George Washington was blistered, bled four times, given calomel as a purgative, and tartar emetic to make him vomit. He had eight pints of blood removed in less than twenty-four hours. This was an overwhelming amount for such a short period of time, and this "heroic treatment" is thought to have hastened his death, which occurred on December 14, 1799. These dramatic techniques, however, were typical for the time and commonly used well into the second half of the nineteenth century. Today it is thought that Washington was probably suffering from a *streptococcus* infection or possibly from diphtheria.

4. Chuinard, Eldong G. *Only One Man Died: The Medical Aspects of the Lewis & Clark Expedition*. Glendale: Arthur Clark, 1979.

5. See the glossary at the back of this book for explanations of medical terminology; see Appendix A for a list of common nineteenth-century medicines and their uses.

6. Ambrose, Stephen E. *Undaunted Courage*. New York: Simon & Schuster, 1996, p. 89.

7. Ibid., 295.

8. Parkman, *The Oregon Trail*, 268.

9. Gardner, *The Domestic Physician*, 79.

10. Ibid., 85.

11. One well-documented case in Europe was that of the Devils of Loudon. In 1632, the prioress, Sister Jeanne, and several of the nuns at the Ursuline Convent in Loudun, France, claimed that their bodies were possessed by demons. After several unsuccessful attempts to drive out the devils, they were finally "exorcised" when the chief priest ordered that each woman receive a large enema of holy water. For a full account, see Huxley, Aldous, *The Devils of Loudun*, New York: Harper & Row, 1952. This was apparently not an unusual form of treatment for exorcism. Another case of demonic possession in France was reportedly treated with success by the same primitive means in Paris in 1854.

12. Gardner, *The Domestic Physician*, 115–116.

13. For further explanation of the confusion between hysteria, chlorosis, and neurasthenia, and their changing meanings and treatments, see Maines, *Technology*, 21–42; and Dixon, Laurinda S. *Some Penetrating Insights: The Imagery of Enemas in Art. Art Journal*, Fall 1993.

Chapter Two

1. When the Revolutionary War started in 1775, approximately 10 percent of the practicing doctors in the original thirteen colonies had a medical degree that resulted from formal training; the rest had been trained by the apprentice system.

237

2. Carden, W.D., *Nineteenth Century Physicians in Clear Creek County, Colorado, 1865–1895.* Master's Thesis, Yale University, 1968.

3. See Appendix B for the typical contents of a physician's medical kit.

4. Hertzler, *The Horse and Buggy Doctor*, 109.

5. The average price for a doctor visit in Colorado did not change substantially from 1860 to 1895, as the following chart shows.

Date	Office visit	Delivery	Minor surgery	Major surgery
1860	$2	$25–200	$10–25	$ 50–500
1895	$5	$20– 50	$ 5–10	$100–500

Data adapted from Shrikes (1986).

6. Enss, *The Doctor Wore Petticoats*, 53.

7. During the Civil War, Union forces lost 360,222 men. Out of this total, 110,070 died from battlefield injuries, and 224,586 died from disease. The commonest killers were diarrhea and dysentery, followed by malaria. During one campaign, the Union Army reported that out of a force of 52,178 men, 12,284 (24 percent) were laid low with diarrhea and dysentery, and 3,866 (7 percent) had contracted malaria. A full 25 percent of the force was on the sick list with wounds and various diseases.

The following lists the soldiers in the Union Army during the Civil War who suffered from various diseases, compiled from 5,825,480 cases that reported for sick call.

Disease	Number of Cases	Number of Deaths
Diarrhea or dysentery	1,585,236	37,794
Gonorrhea	95,833	6
Syphilis	73,382	123
Typhoid	73,368	27,050
Malarial fever	49,871	4,059
Scurvy	30,714	383
Delirium Tremens (alcoholism)	3,744	450

Data adapted from Wilbur (1998).

Chapter Three

1. The name "miasma" comes from the Greek word for pollution.

2. Burros are still allowed to freely roam the streets of Cripple Creek, Colorado, in the summer in an attempt to recreate the early atmosphere of the mining town during its boom days.

3. Severe fires in mountain mining towns, such as the one that burned Crested Butte, Colorado, on February 8, 1963, can be worsened by cold weather. The temperature dropped to -40° F, and firemen found that the brand new fire hydrant system had frozen solid.

4. Hertzler, *The Horse and Buggy Doctor*, 105.

5. *The Household*, Vol. 7, No. 1, January 1874, p. 4.

6. Morgan, Lael. *Good Time Girls.* Kenmore: Epicenter Press, 1998, pp. 227–228.

7. Alkali was a generic name for strong salts of sodium and potassium that were poisonous if they were present in high enough concentration in the water.

8. Even today, law enforcement officers are known to have a higher incidence of heart disease and colon cancer than the general population due to poor diet resulting from their working conditions.

Chapter Four

1. Cholera first entered England in 1831, via the port city of Newcastle, on a ship from India. One major outbreak in 1848–9 cost 55,000 lives. Another serious epidemic occurred in 1853–4 in London. In the first few days of the outbreak, over 300 cases were diagnosed, with another 200 following over the next few weeks. The source of the outbreak was finally traced by physician John Snow to a shallow well on Broad Street (now Broadwick Street) that served as a communal water supply. Further investigation showed that a nearby privy vault was leaking into the well and contaminating the water. It was later discovered that a young baby in the area had died of cholera a few weeks previously, and that her feces, while she was ill, had been disposed of in the leaking privy. This started a circular process that continued from the sewer to drinking water to people, then back to the sewer again in a vicious cycle. As early as 1849 Snow had shown that cholera was a water-borne disease, and his investigation in Broad Street proved his point conclusively.

2. Parkman, *The Oregon Trail*, 46.

3. Ibid., 99.

4. Ibid., 317–318.

5. Hertzler, *The Horse and Buggy Doctor*, 1–2.

6. Gardner, *The Domestic Physician*, 88.

7. Malaria is transmitted by female mosquitoes, because only the females bite and suck blood. Female mosquitoes require a blood meal in order for their eggs to mature before they are laid. The males feed on plant juices.

8. As a curious side note to malaria, the sickle cell trait among black Africans gave them some immunity against *vivax* malaria, a characteristic that made them ideal workers as slaves on plantations in the mosquito-infested Caribbean and southern United States.

9. Unfortunately, some pioneers looking for wild onions mistakenly dug up the bulbs of the death-camas plant, which looked similar to the wild onion but which was poisonous. Even today, death-camas is one of the most frequent killers of domestic sheep, which eat the plants readily. As author Gregory Tilfort succinctly put it, "Do not mess with this plant." An extract from the poisonous root was put into streams by American Indians to immobilize fish to make them easier to catch.

10. Hertzler, *The Horse and Buggy Doctor*, 5.

11. Angear, J.H. "Consumption Primarily a Nerve Disease," *Journal of the American Medical Association*, 20: 558–560, May 20, 1893.

12. When French emperor Napoleon invaded Russia in 1812, his troops suffered a devastating typhus epidemic that decimated almost all of his army of 600,000 men.

13. This was not a new idea. In Europe, during the Black Plague epidemics of the 1300s, bells were rung and guns were fired to "break up" the air. As with yellow fever later, these efforts were to no avail.

Chapter Five

1. This was at a time when one authority gravely pronounced that women who tried to educate themselves would take on male characteristics, which included sterility, the growth of facial hair, and shriveling of the female reproductive organs.

2. Hershey, E.P. "Modes of Infection," *Colorado Medical Journal*, 6: 275 (1900).

3. Gonorrhea is described in the Old Testament, in the Book of Leviticus, along with cautions to refrain from having sex, which would transmit the disease to other people. In 1976, one million cases of gonorrhea were reported to the U.S. Public Health Service, most of them occurring in the category of fifteen to twenty-nine year-olds. The disease peaked in the period 1975–1980, when the incidence was 450 per 100,000 population, and has since declined. Today, gonorrhea is second only to the common cold in the incidence of communicable diseases.

4. Estimates are as high as 75 percent of Western prostitutes caught some form of venereal disease at some time in their career. Repeated and prolonged exposure to gonorrhea made many prostitutes sterile, thus unknowingly freeing them from the burdens of pregnancy.

5. Eliason et al., *Surgical Nursing*, 554.

6. The chemical composition of Salvarsan 606 was dioxy-diamino-arsenobenzol-dihydrochloride. In 1917, fears that supplies of Salvarsan from Germany would be cut off due to the outbreak of World War I caused American manufacturers to begin making a similar drug called Arsphenamine. The names of the two drugs are often used interchangeably.

7. *California Daily News*, April 12, 1843.

8. Stockham, Alice. *Tokology: A Book for Every Woman*. London: L.N. Fowler, 1900, p. 31.

Chapter Six

1. In 1825, James Hamilton in England reported using purging for such diverse conditions as typhus, scarlet fever, emaciation, hysteria, tetanus, chlorosis (see the glossary for the dual meaning of chlorosis), and St. Vitus dance (a nervous disease characterized by involuntary muscular twitching, now called chorea).

2. The idea of ridding the body of toxic substances was not new. Greek physician Herodotus (484–425 B.C.), who traveled extensively in ancient Egypt, noted that the Egyptians fasted and used purgatives, enemas, and emetics for three consecutive days each month in the belief that disease came from the food they consumed.

3. Whorton, *Inner Hygiene*, 116.

4. The term "physic" is also an archaic

general name used for medical science or the art of healing.

5. For a more detailed account of the extensive treatments that the human digestive system was subjected to in the late nineteenth century, see Gant, *Constipation and Intestinal Obstruction*, chapters 20–27.

6. In France in the 1770s, druggists sold a purgative pill called "a perpetual pill," that was made from antimony. The pill was swallowed and produced an irritating purgative action as it passed unchanged through the digestive tract. The pill could later be recovered, washed, and used again and again. Perpetual pills were treated as family heirlooms, and "after passing through one generation were passed on to the next," so to speak.

7. Ambrose, Stephen E. *Undaunted Courage*. New York: Simon & Schuster, 1996, p. 90.

8. Hertzler, *The Horse and Buggy Doctor*, 231.

9. The legal sale of narcotic drugs, such as opium, cocaine, and morphine, over the counter ended with the Harrison Narcotic Act of 1914.

10. By the early 1700s, the British were importing large amounts of tea, silk, and porcelain from China, creating an undesired outflow of silver from the British Treasury. The equalizer turned out to be opium. Working against Chinese resistance, the British-based East India Company sold massive quantities of opium grown in India to China in the late 1700s and early 1800s in an attempt to force a balance in the exchange of trade. In 1858 the Treaty of Tientsin legalized this opium traffic and helped to spread addiction.

11. Green, *The Light of the Home*, 140.

12. These substances were called alkaloids because they turned litmus paper blue, which is the sign of an alkaline chemical substance.

13. In a similar manner, methadone is used today to wean addicts from heroin dependence because methadone addiction, which is similar to morphine dependence, is easier to cure than heroin addiction.

14. Child, *The Family Nurse*, 102.

15. For a collection of reports from newspapers and periodicals on this unexplained phenomenon, see Fort, Charles H. *The Books of Charles Fort*. New York: Henry Holt, 1941, pp. 656–7, 661–3, 927–30.

16. Utley, Robert M., ed. *Life in Custer's Cavalry: Diaries and Letters of Albert and Jennie Barnitz, 1867–1868*. Lincoln: University of Nebraska Press, 1977, p. 139.

17. Most drugs, even prescription drugs that are considered to be safe when prescribed and used under medical supervision, have the potential for harmful side effects and interaction with other drugs, a reality that is not perceived by those indulging in today's abusive practice of "pharming," which is the indiscriminate mixing and ingesting of prescription drugs to experiment with their possible mind-altering effects.

18. In Europe, in the Middle Ages, accidental ergot poisoning from consuming moldy rye resulted in a disease called "St. Anthony's Fire" or "Hellfire." Constriction of the blood supply in the extremities, due to eating the mold, caused gangrene to develop and the fingers and toes dropped off without bleeding.

19. Parkman, *The Oregon Trail*, 95–6.

20. Russel, W. Kerr. *Colonic Irrigation*. Edinburgh: E. & S. Livingstone, 1932, page 6.

21. Treating drowning victims by treating their bowels was apparently a common practice in the mid–1800s. In 1852, *The Ladies' Indispensible Assistant* recommended an enema of spirits of turpentine to revive those who had nearly drowned.

Chapter Seven

1. Manuals for the home treatment of medical conditions were widespread among the colonists of America. One example of an early manual was *Every Man His Own Doctor*, which was published in 1734 by John Tennent.

2. Child, *The Family Nurse*, 3.

3. Indeed, approximately 40 percent of the drugs used in modern medicine are derived from plants.

4. C.S. Rafinesque (1828), quoted in Meyer, *American Folk Medicine*, 147.

5. This may actually have been effective. Soap concocted with coal tar derivatives was still available as an anti-dandruff shampoo as late as the 1950s.

6. Hutchinson, *Ladies' Indispensible Assistant*, 15.

7. Ibid., 16.

8. Both jalap and ipecac originated in the New World, where they were used as a purge and emetic, respectively, by Indians of Central and South America. Both plants were taken back to Europe to be used as a medicine by early white explorers.

9. Hutchinson, *Ladies' Indispensible Assistant*, 16.

10. Ibid., 56.

Chapter Eight

1. Hertzler, *The Horse and Buggy Doctor*, 7.

2. Ibid., p. 6–7.

3. Ignatz Semmelweis died in 1865, ironically after a wound on his finger, acquired during an autopsy, became infected by the same bacteria that he had identified as causing deaths from childbirth fever.

4. Hertzler, *The Horse and Buggy Doctor*, 118.

5. Carbolic acid is toxic, caustic, and has a powerful odor, all of which must have made its use daunting for the surgeon. Another disadvantage was that it also burned the surgeon's skin.

6. Hertzler, *The Horse and Buggy Doctor*, 9.

7. The operating theater at St. Thomas Hospital in London in the 1800s was located in a wooden garret well away from the patient wards, so that the screams of the individual undergoing surgery could not be heard by patients in the hospital. The term operating "theater" came into use because early operating rooms were constructed like theaters for stage performances. They were packed with medical students seated in ascending rows around the operating table, each student trying to get a good view of the surgeon who was operating, in order to learn the newest techniques.

8. And indeed it has retained its popularity. Breathing nitrous oxide for the "high" effects obtained was popular at so-called "Rave Parties" in the late 1980s and early 1990s.

9. When the author was a small boy, he had the experience of having a deep gash in his leg sewn up without the use of any local anesthetic to dull the pain. Even though this was a relatively minor procedure, he can understand the appalling pain that patients who underwent major surgery must have felt.

10. Hertzler, *The Horse and Buggy Doctor*, 237.

11. James Simpson was eventually knighted by Queen Victoria for his contributions to the relief of pain.

12. Abbott, *We Pointed Them North*, 214–5.

13. Burns, *Tombstone*, 63.

14. Similar probes were still standard issue in army field surgery kits up to the time of World War II.

Chapter Nine

1. Phthisis is an older medical term for tuberculosis (consumption). Black phthisis was the name for lung disease in coal miners, resulting from inhaling coal dust.

2. A vertical hole in the ground is called a *shaft*. A horizontal opening at ground level is technically named an *adit* or *portal*. A horizontal working space underground is a *drift*. A *tunnel* is technically a horizontal passage that is open at both ends. A large underground cavity formed by the removal of ore is called a *stope*.

3. Fulminate of mercury was used in the percussion cap of percussion revolvers and rifles. When the trigger was pulled, a sharp blow from the hammer of the gun ignited the percussion cap, which in turn ignited the main powder charge in the breech of the gun.

4. The modern short, wide snowshoes of today were not in use at the time. What the miners of the late 1800s called "snowshoes," "Norwegian shoes," or "snowskates" were what are today called cross-country skis. These skis were ten to eleven feet long and three to four inches wide. Instead of two short, modern ski poles, a single long, lightweight pole was used to provide balance and assist in forward motion.

5. Blasting caps from the mining era are still found around old mine sites today. Over the years they have typically become very unstable and people picking them up or accidentally standing on them while investigating historic mine sites can lose fingers and toes.

6. Lathrop, *Little Engines and Big Men*, 34.

7. "Free gold" is gold that is found in its natural state as dust particles or nuggets of pure gold, as opposed to gold that occurs in complex ores, such as sylvanite and calaverite, which require chemical treatment to extract the gold from the other chemicals.

8. Sodium cyanide is so poisonous that it was used for executions in the gas chamber. The cyanide leaching process is still used today in large open-pit mining operations to

extract minuscule amounts of pure gold from waste rock.

9. In the 1970s the author met a rodeo cowboy in his forties who had suffered so many falls from horse and bull riding, and broken so many bones, that he was permanently confined to bed in a nursing home and could hardly move.

10. Abbott, *We Pointed Them North*, 63.

11. Lathrop, *Little Engines and Big Men*, 67.

12. Pitkin, *Review*, July 20, 1882.

13. *Gunnison Weekly Review*, July 22, 1882.

14. *Buena Vista Colorado Democrat*, May 29, 1895.

15. Lathrop, *Little Engines and Big Men*, 66.

16. Abbott, Dan. *Colorado Midland Railway*. Denver: Sundance Publications, 1989, p. 174.

17. Lathrop, *Little Engines and Big Men*, 79.

Chapter Ten

1. The Victorians were a particularly morbid society and were obsessed with death and disease, in part because they were surrounded by both in their daily lives. Hugely popular amusement attractions were the so-called "anatomical museums," which displayed grisly diseased and malformed organs for public viewing and titillation under the guise of "scientific education." Models and displays in these museums that dealt with reproductive functions and diseased reproductive organs were particularly popular because sex was a subject that was taboo in polite Victorian society.

2. Bergersen, *Pharmacology in Nursing*, 239.

3. Sanders, *Modern Methods in Nursing*, 347.

4. Child, *The Family Nurse*, 4.

5. Holbrook, *The Golden Age of Quackery*, 32.

6. From newspaper advertising for Paine's Celery Compound, 1888.

7. Armstrong, *The Great American Medicine Show*, 162.

8. Similar patent medicine shows can be found today in parts of Asia.

9. Advertisement for the Lydia Pinkham Company in *The Standard Delineator*, February 1896.

10. Queen Victoria of England was found to have a displaced uterus only after she died.

11. In direct current systems, such as batteries, the voltage source maintains a constant polarity and the current flows from the positive electrode to the negative. In alternating current systems, the polarity of the voltage alternates, or reverses, a certain number of times each second. In today's homes, the alternations occur at sixty times per second, or sixty Hertz (abbreviated Hz).

12. The use of electrotherapy to relieve pain is the basis of today's Transcutaneous Electrical Nerve Stimulation (TENS) devices, which send a small electric current through the skin. These devices can be very effective in cases of intractable pain, such as inoperable back pain.

13. It is possible that the popularity of such treatments may have been due to pleasurable side-effects, as ejaculation was claimed to be a common side-effect of rectally administered electrotherapy. Rectal electrostimulation is commonly used on bulls and stallions to produce sperm for artificial insemination. In 1948, and again in 1984, doctors with the Veteran's Administration tried to gather sperm, using similar techniques, from veterans with spinal cord injuries so that they might father children. Further details may be found in Warner, Harold, et al., "Electrostimulation of Erection and Ejaculation and Collection of Semen in Spinal Cord Injured Humans," *Journal of Rehabilitation Research and Development*, Vol. 23, No. 3, 1986, pp 21–31. See also Maines, *Technology*, chapter four.

14. *Silver City Independent*, June 14, 1921.

15. As a curious footnote to blue light, current experiments in Japan indicate that blue lighting may lead to a decrease in the number of suicides by jumping in front of trains in railroad stations. Professor Tsuneo Suzuki, at Keio University in Japan, feels that blue lighting may produce a calming effect in people; however, he also adds that it is too early to draw any conclusions. In Nara, Japan, in 2005, and in Glasgow, Scotland, the use of blue street lighting seems to be linked to a decrease in crime in neighborhoods with these lights.

Chapter Eleven

1. When the author was a small boy, the use of slow-speed dental drills and a lack of dental anesthetics was common. Having un-

dergone this type of dental procedure, he can sympathize with dental patients in the Old West.

2. The name "rubber" was initially applied to the soft, sticky sap that came from the rubber tree that grows in tropical countries. Charles Goodyear developed a process to cure India rubber by heating it with sulfur to create the soft latex rubber used for rubber gloves and other medical devices. If the sulfur process was carried to the extreme, the rubber became solid, and the resulting hard material was called "hard rubber" or "vulcanite."

Chapter Twelve

1. Enema syringes made from animal bladders were in use by American Indians before contact with Europeans. They were used to treat constipation, diarrhea, and hemorrhoids. This practice may have originated in South America in pre–Columbian times. South American Indians were known to have made hollow ball syringes for enemas from the sap of the rubber tree. Pottery found in Mayan ruins in Central America depicts the use of enemas during religious rituals that are thought to have contained hallucinogenic substances. The Aztec used syringes to inject wine. South American Indians used rubber syringes to inject cohoba, a type of snuff with narcotic properties that was prepared from the pods of the *acacia niopo* plant. Both the Catauixis Indians and the Mura Indians of the Upper Amazon basin of Brazil ground the pods into a powder, mixed it with water, and injected the resulting solution as an enema, using the leg bone of the tuyuyu bird (wood ibis). The active ingredient in the mixture was *serotonin*, a substance that impaired the perception of time and space. The Indians felt that it cleared the vision and made the senses more alert during hunting expeditions.

2. Supposedly, yarrow was used by Achilles, the Greek hero of the Trojan War, to cure the wounds of his soldiers after battle.

3. Both the skunk cabbage and the Indian turnip (also known as Jack-in-the pulpit) were later found to have effective medicinal properties and were eventually accepted into both *The Pharmacopeia of the United States of America* (the USP), the listing of approved medicinal agents, and the *National Formulary*, which is essentially a supplement to the USP, sponsored by the American Pharmaceutical Association.

4. Many of these diseases had their origins in the close association during the Middle Ages of European populations with domestic animals, such as cows and horses, who passed on many diseases that appeared in mutated form in man.

Bibliography

Abbott, Edward C., and Helena H. Smith. *We Pointed Them North*. New York: Farrar & Rinehart, 1939.

Ackerknecht, Erwin H. *A Short History of Medicine*. Baltimore: Johns Hopkins University Press, 1982.

Adams, George W. *Doctors in Blue*. New York: Henry Schuman, 1952.

Agnew, Jeremy. *Brides of the Multitude: Prostitution in the Old West*. Lake City: Western Reflections Publishing, 2008.

_____. *Life of a Soldier on the Western Frontier*. Missoula: Mountain Press Publishing, 2008.

Anderson, Ann. *Snake Oil, Hustlers and Hambones: The American Medicine Show*. Jefferson, NC: McFarland, 2000.

Armstrong, David, and Elizabeth M. Armstrong. *The Great American Medicine Show*. New York: Prentice Hall, 1991.

Bad Hand, Howard P. *Native American Healing*. Chicago: Keats Publishing, 2002.

Bergersen, Betty S., and Elsie E. Krug. *Pharmacology in Nursing*. St. Louis: C.V. Mosby, 1966.

Blair, Edward. *Leadville: Colorado's Magic City*. Boulder: Pruett Publishing, 1980.

Bloom, Khaled J. *The Mississippi Valley's Great Yellow Fever Epidemic of 1878*. Baton Rouge: Louisiana State University Press, 1993.

Bollet, Alfred J. *Civil War Medicine*. Tucson: Galen Press, 2002.

Brady, George S. *Materials Handbook*. New York: McGraw-Hill, 1963.

Breeden, James O., ed. *Medicine in the West*. Manhattan: Sunflower University Press, 1982.

Burns, Walter N. *Tombstone*. New York: Doubleday, 1927.

Byrne, Bernard J. *A Frontier Army Surgeon*. Cranford: Allen Printing, 1935.

Calhoun, Mary H. *Medicine Show: Conning People and Making Them Like It*. New York: Harper & Row, 1976.

Child, Lydia M. *The Family Nurse: or Companion of the American Frugal Housewife*. Boston: Charles J. Hendee, 1837.

Clendening, Logan. *Behind the Doctor*. New York: Alfred A. Knopf, 1933.

Cornell, Virginia. *Doc Susie*. Tucson: Manifest Publications, 1991.

Craig, Robert G., and Floyd A. Peyton. *Restorative Dental Materials*. St. Louis: C.V. Mosby, 1975.

Craighead, John J., Frank C. Craighead, Jr., and Ray J. Davis. *A Field Guide to Rocky Mountain Wildflowers*. Boston: Houghton Mifflin, 1963.

Dale, Edward E. *Frontier Ways*. Austin: University of Texas Press, 1959.

Davis, Lucille. *Medicine in the American West*. New York: Scholastic, 2001.

De la Peña, Carolyn T. *The Body Electric: How Strange Machines Built the Modern American*. New York: New York University Press, 2003.

Denney, Robert E. *Civil War Medicine: Care and Comfort of the Wounded*. New York: Sterling, 1994.

Douglas, William A. *A History of Dentistry in Colorado, 1859–1959*. Boulder: Johnson Publishing, 1959.

Dunlop, Richard. *Doctors of the American Frontier*. Garden City: Doubleday, 1965.

Eliason, E.L., L.K. Ferguson, and Evelyn M. Farrand. *Surgical Nursing*. Philadelphia: J.B. Lippincott, 1940.

Enss, Chris. *The Doctor Wore Petticoats*. Guilford: TwoDot, 2006.

Evans & Wormull. *Illustrated Catalogue of Surgical Instruments*. London: Wm. Dawson & Sons, 1876.

Frexinos, Jacques. *L'Art de Purger*. Paris: Editions Louis Pariente, 1997.

Gant, Samuel G. *Constipation and Intestinal Obstruction*. Philadelphia: W.B. Saunders, 1909.

Gardiner, Charles F. *Doctor at Timberline*. Caldwell: Caxton Printers, 1938.

Gardner, Marlin, and Benjamin H. Aylworth. *The Domestic Physician and Family Assistant*. Cooperstown: H. and E. Phinney, 1836.

Green, Harvey. *The Light of the Home*. New York: Pantheon Books, 1983.

Groh, George W. *Gold Fever: Being a True Account, Both Horrifying and Hilarious of the Art of Healing (So-Called) During the California Gold Rush*. New York: William Morrow, 1966.

Hall, Thomas B. *Medicine on the Santa Fe Trail*. Dayton: Morningside Bookshop, 1971.

Heatherley, Ana N. *Healing Plants: A Medicinal Guide to Native North American Plants and Herbs*. New York: Lyons Press, 1998.

Hertzler, Arthur E. *The Horse and Buggy Doctor*. Lincoln: University of Nebraska Press, 1970.

Holbrook, Stewart H. *The Golden Age of Quackery*. New York: Macmillan, 1959.

Holmes, King K., P. Fredrick Sparling, Per-Anders Mårdh, et al. *Sexually Transmitted Diseases*. New York: McGraw-Hill, 1999.

Hutchinson, E. *Ladies' Indispensible Assistant*. New York: (publisher unlisted), 1852.

Jones, Billy M. *Health Seekers in the Southwest, 1817–1900*. Norman: University of Oklahoma Press, 1967.

Karolevitz, Robert F. *Doctors of the Old West*. Seattle: Superior Publishing, 1967.

Kuz, Julian E., and Bradley P. Bengtson. *Orthopaedic Injuries of the Civil War*. Kennesaw: Kennesaw Mountain Press, 1996.

Lathrop, Gilbert A. *Little Engines and Big Men*. Caldwell: Caxton Printers, 1954.

Maines, Rachel P. *The Technology of Orgasm*. Baltimore: Johns Hopkins University Press, 1999.

Marks, Geoffrey, and William K. Beatty. *The Story of Medicine in America*. New York: Scribner's, 1973.

McIntosh, Elaine N. *The Lewis & Clark Expedition*. Sioux Falls: Center for Western Studies, 2003.

Meyer, Clarence. *American Folk Medicine*. New York: Thomas Y. Crowell, 1973.

Miller, Brandon M. *Just What the Doctor Ordered: The History of American Medicine*. Minneapolis: Lerner Publications, 1997.

Moore, Michael. *Medicinal Plants of the Mountain West*. Santa Fe: Museum of New Mexico Press, 1979.

Mulcahy, Robert. *Diseases: Finding the Cure*. Minneapolis: Oliver Press, 1996.

_____. *Medical Technology: Inventing the Instruments*. Minneapolis: Oliver Press, 1997.

Nester, Eugene W., et al. *Microbiology: A Human Perspective, 4th Edition*. Boston: McGraw-Hill, 2004.

Parkman, Francis. *The Oregon Trail*. Garden City: Doubleday, 1946.

Pfeiffer, Carl J. *The Art and Practice of Western Medicine in the Early Nineteenth Century*. Jefferson, NC: McFarland, 1985.

Pierce, R.V. *The People's Common Sense Medical Advisor in Plain English*. Buffalo: World's Dispensary Printing, 1895.

Poling-Kempes, Lesley. *The Harvey Girls: Women Who Opened the West*. New York: Marlowe, 1991.

Porter, Roy. *Blood & Guts: A Short History of Medicine*. New York: W.W. Norton, 2003.

_____, ed. *The Cambridge History of Medicine*. New York: Cambridge University Press, 2006.

Ritchie, David, and Fred Israel. *Health and Medicine*. New York: Chelsea House Publishers, 1995.

Rutkow, Ira M. *Bleeding Blue and Gray*. New York: Random House, 2005.

Ryan, Frank. *The Forgotten Plague*. Boston: Little, Brown, 1992.

Sanders, Georgiana J. *Modern Methods in Nursing*. Philadelphia: W.B. Saunders, 1917.

Savage, Douglas J. *Civil War Medicine*. Philadelphia: Chelsea House Publishers, 2000.

Shrikes, Robert H. *Rocky Mountain Medicine*. Boulder: Johnson Books, 1986.

Shryock, Richard H. *Medicine in America: Historical Essays*. Baltimore: Johns Hopkins Press, 1966.

Smith, Duane A., and Ronald C. Brown. *No One Ailing Except a Physician: Medicine in the Mining West, 1848–1919*. Boulder: University Press of Colorado, 2001.

Steele, Volney. *Bleed, Blister and Purge: A History of Medicine on the American Frontier*. Missoula: Mountain Press Publishing, 2005.

Straubing, Harold E. *In Hospital and Camp.* Harrisburg: Stackpole Books, 1993.

Summers, Leigh. *Bound to Please: A History of the Victorian Corset.* Oxford: Berg, 2001.

Sutcliffe, Jenny, and Nancy Duin. *A History of Medicine.* London: Morgan Samuel Editions, 1992.

Taber, Clarence W. *Taber's Cyclopedic Medical Dictionary.* 10th ed. Philadelphia: F.A. Davis, 1965.

Teller, Michael E. *The Tuberculosis Movement.* New York: Greenwood Press, 1988.

Tilfort, Gregory L. *Edible and Medicinal Plants of the West.* Missoula: Mountain Press Publishing, 1997.

Toledo-Pereyra, Luis H. *A History of American Medicine from the Colonial Period to the Early Twentieth Century.* Lewiston: Edward Mellen Press, 2006.

Van Steenwyk, Elizabeth. *Frontier Fever: The Silly, Superstitious — and Sometimes Sensible — Medicine of the Pioneers.* New York: Walker Publishing, 1995.

Vogel, Virgil J. *American Indian Medicine.* Norman: University of Oklahoma Press, 1970.

Warren, David J. *Old Medical and Dental Instruments.* Princes Risborough: Shire Publications, 1994.

Watkins, Arthur L. *A Manual of Electrotherapy.* Philadelphia: Lea & Febiger, 1958.

Webb, Gerald B. *René Théophile Hyacinthe Laënnec.* New York: Paul B. Hoeber, 1928.

Whorton, James C. *Inner Hygiene.* New York: Oxford University Press, 2000.

Wilbur, C. Keith. *Antique Medical Instruments.* Atglen, PA: Schiffer Publishing, 1987.

_____. *Civil War Medicine, 1861–1865.* Old Saybrook, CT: Globe Pequot Press, 1998.

_____ *Revolutionary Medicine, 1700–1800.* Old Saybrook, CT: Globe Pequot Press, 1980.

Williams, Guy. *The Age of Miracles: Medicine and Surgery in the Nineteenth Century.* Chicago: Academy Chicago Publishers, 1981.

Index

Numbers in **bold italics** indicate pages with photographs.